AN ILLUSTR

101
medicinal herbs

STEVEN FOSTER

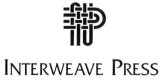

INTERWEAVE PRESS

To the teachers who profoundly impacted my life:
Sister Mildred Barker, Les Eastman, Dr. Shiu Ying Hu,
Brother Theodore Johnson, and Gail Scammon

Acknowledgments

This book could not have been published without the vision, assistance, and recommendations of many behind-the-scenes contributors. First, I thank Mark Blumenthal for his close review of the finished manuscript, for contributing the foreword, and for his wisdom and counsel during the last twenty years. Mary Pat Boian provided suggestions, research materials, advice, and a careful eye to editing before the manuscript was submitted. Thanks to my assistant Kim Seymour and my able graphics advisor, Jonathan Marshall, for their contributions. Ellen Miller—thank you for your generous and invaluable help and support in pushing this project forward. A special thanks to Linda Ligon and Logan Chamberlain at Interweave Press for the vision. I am grateful to Don Brown of Natural Products Research Consultants for providing some hard-to-find original research materials. Finally, thanks to my son Colin and daughter Abbey for dragging me out of the office when "You shouldn't be working."

—Steven Foster
Fayetteville, Arkansas, April 1998

Cover design, Bren Frisch
All photography, Steven Foster

Text copyright 1998, Steven Foster
All photography copyright 1998, Steven Foster

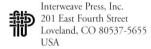
Interweave Press, Inc.
201 East Fourth Street
Loveland, CO 80537-5655
USA

The information in this book should not be used as a substitute for advice from a qualified health-care practitioner. Dosage information is provided as a general guide. Some medicinal herbs may cause allergic reactions in susceptible individuals, and others may not be right to use for particular health conditions.

Library of Congress Cataloging-in-Publication Data

Foster, Steven, 1957-
  101 Medicinal herbs: an illustrated guide / by Steven Foster.
    p.   cm.
  Includes bibliographical references and index.
  ISBN 1-883010-61-6 ISBN 1-883010-51-9 (pbk.)
    1. Herbs — Therapeutic use — Handbooks, manuals, etc. 2. Materia medica, Vegetable — Handbooks, manuals, etc. I. Title.
  RM666.H33F669 1998
  615`.321 — dc21   98-28056
                                                                      CIP

Printed in the United States of America
First printing: 5M:898:RRD
Second printing: 6M:799:RRD

Foreword

As the fastest-growing segment of the dietary supplement industry, herbs are no longer the domain of health-food stores, mail-order houses, and multilevel marketers. They are big business in places where big business is done—drugstores, supermarkets, and mass merchandisers. Herb sales in 1997 were 80 percent higher than 1996 sales in these outlets; total U.S. sales are expected to reach $4 billion in 1998. Wall Street Investment bankers have identified the herb market as the biggest investment opportunity since the advent of the high-tech industry 25 years ago.

The World Health Organization recognizes that herb use is increasing; it estimates that about 80 percent of the world's population still depends on traditional medicine for primary health care, and every form of traditional medicine uses herbs. In most countries, herbs are not "alternative" or "unconventional" but integral to the dominant health-care system. World herb sales were estimated at $12.4 billion in 1993, not counting Africa, South America, and parts of Asia (for which figures were not available). About half these sales were in western Europe and half again in Germany alone.

As the herb movement grows, products proliferate, and millions of Americans turn to them for health care and self-care. For those who may be exploring herbs for the first time, Steven Foster has written a book based on his respect for the traditions of the past and his knowledge of contemporary scientific research. He brings to this task a fervent love of plants, a thorough grasp of the botanical and clinical literature, and a selection of his exquisite herb photographs.

I first met Steven in 1978 at a "Boston Tea Party" staged in protest of the U. S. Food and Drug Administration ban on sassafras tea. The sassafras bark pitched over the sides of the Boston Tea Party Ship and Museum had been collected by Steven, then a young herbalist from Maine. We met again that year at the second annual Herb Trade Association Symposium on Herbs, a seminal event that brought backwoods herbalists, dropout herbalists, manufacturers of the budding herb industry, pharmacognosists, and ethnobotanists together for the first time. Almost twenty years have passed, the herb movement has blossomed and flourished, and Steven has emerged as one of the most knowledgeable and lucid writers in the field. He has published countless articles and numerous books, including the first on echinacea, which has established him as a leader among responsible echinacea promoters and educators.

In the sixteenth century, Paracelsus coined the term "essential oil" for the volatile oils that he believed represented the quintessence of many plants. Today, Steven Foster's writing and photography represent the quintessence of modern herbal literature.

—Mark Blumenthal
Founder and Executive Director
American Botanical Council
Editor, *HerbalGram*

Contents

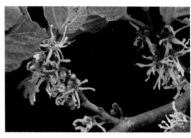
Witch Hazel

Medicinal Herbs

Cayenne

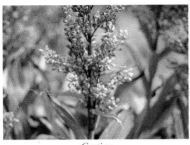

Gentian

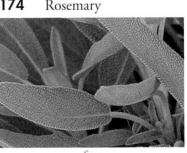

Sage

Introduction

Herbs have been used for healing throughout history, and even now they play a part in the modern, high-tech world of medicine: About 25 percent of today's pharmaceutical drugs contain chemicals derived from plants. Researchers continue to examine plants and study the history of herbalism in hope of discovering new drugs for cancer, AIDS, and even the common cold.

Because I'm a skeptic at heart, if someone says a herb is good for this or that, I say, "Prove it."

Herbal healing, however, goes far beyond using isolated chemicals from plants for healing. In this, contemporary herbalism owes much to European phytomedicine (literally, plant medicine), which uses preparations from an entire plant or from its root, leaf, flower, or fruit. Thus, compounds such as menthol (from peppermint) or digitoxin (from foxglove) are not considered phytomedicines, but a cup of chamomile tea made from the dried flower is. Herbalists believe that using the whole plant or its major parts offers benefits more subtle and powerful than using only isolated chemicals.

In this century, Germany has led the way in confirming Western herbalism's traditional uses of herbs and discovering new, effective uses as well. Herbs undergo rigorous study; those approved by Commission E, a group of physicians, herbalists, pharmacists, and other health professionals, may be prescribed and sold as drugs. The commission publishes and distributes papers about the herbs, summarizing the studies and their findings.

The German studies have fueled American interest in healing herbs. More than ever, people are searching for ways to improve their health. Some want natural good health through diet, exercise, and supportive herbs. Others are wary of the side effects and high costs of pharmaceutical drugs and want gentle healing from herbs.

And some are fed up with the restrictions and interference of their health maintenance organizations and want to take charge of their own health.

Herbal medicines are classified as dietary supplements in the United States, and the law restricts the claims manufacturers can make about the herb's healing properties. When such claims are made, the product label must include the following: *This statement has not been evaluated by the Food and Drug Administration. This product is not intended to diagnose, treat, cure, or prevent disease.* Manufacturers must register the claim with the Secretary of Health and Human Services and be fully prepared to back it up with scientific evidence.

As an example, a manufacturer may claim that a garlic product helps reduce cholesterol if the disclaimer is included on the label. Forbidden, however, is the claim that *garlic* helps reduce cholesterol *and thus reduces the risk of heart disease.* People not involved in the manufacture of herbal products can publish scientific information about medicinal herbs.

No wonder it's bewildering to shop for herbs. Health and natural products stores offer dried, powdered, and cut-and-sifted herbs, as well as herbs prepared in tinctures, capsules, tablets, and more. In grocery stores and pharmacies, herbal preparations are often lined up right next to over-the-counter drugs for headaches and cold symptoms. Rarely does store clerk know enough to help you, even if you ask questions. How can you decide what herbs are best for you, and how should herbs be used?

> **Herbalists believe that using the whole plant or its major parts offers benefits more subtle and powerful than using only isolated chemicals.**

This book is a quick reference guide to the 101 herbs most often sold as dietary supplements to support natural health, and it includes both modern scientific information and the history and traditions of herbs. Because I'm a skeptic at heart, if someone says a herb is good for this or that, I say, "Prove it." So I have searched the scientific literature for laboratory or human studies that prove or disprove traditional claims about herbs. Each herb entry contains the following information.

Common and botanical names. The common names of herbs may be charming but confusing, too. Siberian ginseng, for instance, is not a ginseng, or *Panax,* at all, but the root of a shrub, *Eleutherococcus senticosus.* Knowing both botanical and common names of herbs helps you get the best product.

Historical uses. Many herbs have been "tested" for thousands of years as traditional healers have used them to help the sick. These fascinating herbal traditions influence the use of herbs today.

Health conditions and herbal actions. Symptoms and illnesses are listed, along with the helpful actions of the herb. For instance, ginkgo helps age-related memory loss by increasing microcirculation, or blood and oxygen flow, to the tiny blood vessels in the brain.

Forms of the herb typically available. Capsules, tincture, or powder?

Dosages. How much herb should you take, and how often? And for how long? These guidelines help you get started. They are based on Germany's Commission E regulations, industry research, Chinese pharmacy texts, and other authoritative sources.

Cautions. Certain herbs may not be right for you because of allergies, a chronic illness, or drugs you must take. Remember that any substance—natural or man-made—can cause problems for some people.

Guidelines for Selecting Herbs

Because I use herbs one way or another nearly every day, I shop often for them. My plan for using the herbs usually determines what form I select. If I've had trouble sleeping lately and want a calming bedtime tea for a few weeks, I'll probably purchase a couple of handsful of dried chamomile flowers. If I need the tonic properties of Asian ginseng for the long-term, however, I'll likely choose a preparation in a more convenient and concentrated form, such as capsules or tincture. These more expensive herbs are well worth the money.

Each herb entry in this book contains information similar to that found on the labels of herb preparations made by reliable companies. A simple package may be labeled "St.-John's-wort" in big letters, but if the side panel doesn't include the herb's name, or the name is misspelled, or the label lacks dosage information, don't buy it. If the label indicates that the herb product is diluted with fructose (fruit sugar) or other unwanted substances, pass it by.

Instead, look for a St.-John's-wort product labeled to indicate standardization to hypericin, believed to be the active ingredient in St.-John's-wort. Check the dosage information and warnings, such as taking the herb before spending time in the sun. Such a product is

Making your own herbal preparations, however, offers a particular satisfaction and pleasure. These preparations need not be complicated, and they can be as effective as commercial ones.

likely to be backed by a reliable manufacturing company that takes pride in its products.

Guidelines for Preparing and Using Herbs

Because the U. S. system of measurement is far less accurate in small measures than the metric system, the weights of herbs in this book are expressed in grams (g). Nevertheless, you can roughly translate metric measurements into U. S. measurements.

Dry measurements:

5 g = 1 teaspoon of dried, powdered herb
10 g = 2 teaspoons of dried, powdered herb
3 teaspoons = 1 tablespoon = about 1/2 ounce of dried, powdered herb

Fluid measures of herbs are usually expressed in milliliters (ml). One milliliter is one-thousandth of a liter or about one-thirtieth of a fluid ounce. Here are approximate U. S. equivalents.

Fluid measurements:

10 drops = 1 ml = 1/4 teaspoon
50 drops = 5 ml = 1 teaspoon
6 teaspoons = 2 tablespoons = 1 fluid ounce

To keep life simple, I often recommend that you follow the manufacturer's recommended dosages for capsules, tablets, tinctures, and especially standardized products that deliver a certain weight of an extract or chemical component per dose.

Making your own herbal preparations, however, offers a particular satisfaction and pleasure. These preparations need not be complicated, and they can be as effective as commercial ones.

Teas or infusions are simple preparations made from herb flowers, leaves, stems, or fruit. To make a tea, prepare a cup or teapot with the appropriate amount of herb. In a pan, bring water to a boil, remove from heat, and promptly pour water to fill the tea container. Cover the tea and steep for at least fifteen minutes. Strain out the herb if desired and drink the liquid, one cup two or three times daily. Keep tea in the refrigerator for no more than three days.

Decoctions or "herbal soups" are made from the roots, stems, or bark of herbs that do not give up their benefits easily. First chop, grind, or otherwise break the appropriate amount of herb material into small pieces. Bring a quart of water to boil and add the herb; simmer for 30 to 60 minutes or until the water volume is reduced to 2 or 3 cups. Cool, strain, and drink about half a cup of decoction two or three times a day. Refrigerate for no more than three days.

Tinctures, popular and concentrated extracts of herbs, are produced by soaking the herb in alcohol or percolating alcohol through it, thus drawing out the useful constituents. A product label may carry a ratio such as 5:1, meaning that there are five parts of herb by liquid unit of measure to one part of alcohol. A 5:1 tincture is five times as strong as a 1:1 tincture.

As more people use herbs for healing, they must be armed with the facts to make informed choices on purchasing those dietary-supplement products. Much of that information will be found in these pages. A companion volume which will help, you, the consumer, make the best choices in purchasing herb products is *What the Labels Won't Tell You* by Logan Chamberlain, Ph.D. (Interweave Press, 1998).

> **As more people use herbs for healing, they must be armed with the facts to make informed choices on purchasing those dietary-supplement products. Much of that information will be found in these pages.**

Therapeutic Cross-Reference List

The following list is intended as a quick reference guide to symptoms and conditions for which the listed herbs have clinically proven effects. Before using an unfamiliar herb, you should be careful to read the full profile, especially the cautions.

aches and pains	Prickly ash, Rosemary, Willow, Yucca
acne	Tea tree oil, Witch hazel
angina pectoris	Hawthorn, Kudzu
antioxidant	Cayenne, Grapeseed, Schisandra, Turmeric
anxiety	Hops, Kava-kava, Passionflower, Reishi, Skullcap, St.-John's-wort, Valerian
appetite, lack of	Alfalfa, Blessed thistle, Dandelion, Gentian, Hops, Horehound, Rosemary
asthma, mild	Ephedra
atherosclerosis	Bilberry
benign prostatic hyperplasia (BPH)	Pygeum, Saw palmetto, Stinging nettle
bruises	Arnica, Bilberry, Horse chestnut
burns, first degree	Aloe, Calendula
candida	Tea tree oil
colds	Astragalus, Echinacea, Elderberry, Licorice, Marshmallow, Mullein, Plantain, Thyme

congestion	Ephedra, Horehound, Licorice, Marshmallow, Peppermint
congestive heart failure, early stages	Hawthorn
constipation	Cascara sagrada, Flaxseed, Psyllium, Rhubarb, Senna
convalescence	Ginseng
cuts and abrasions	Aloe, Shepherd's purse, St.-John's-wort (external)
depression, mild to moderate	St.-John's-wort (internal)
detoxification	Burdock
diarrhea	Bilberry, Red raspberry leaves White oak, Witch hazel
digestion	Blessed thistle, Boldo, Dandelion, Gentian, Horehound, Rosemary
diuretic	Broom, Burdock, Celery, Dandelion, Horsetail, Juniper, Nopal, Oatstraw, Parsley, Stinging nettle
earache	Mullein
essential fatty acids deficiency	Borage, Evening primrose, Flaxseed
fatigue	Ginseng
fever	Elderberry, Willow
flu	Astragalus, Echinacea, Elderberry, Licorice, Marshmallow, Mullein, Plantain, Thyme

gas, digestive	Horsetail, Lemon balm, Lemon grass
gastrointestinal irritation or inflammation	Boldo, Flaxseed, Slippery elm, Wild yam
gastrointestinal spasms	Fenugreek, Flaxseed, Peppermint
heart arrhythmia	Motherwort
hemorrhoids	Bilberry, Witch hazel
herpes sores	Lemon balm
indigestion	Chamomile, Devil's claw, Fennel, Fenugreek, Gentian, Ginger, Juniper, Marshmallow, Sage, Turmeric
infections, minor	Astragalus, Cat's-claw, Echinacea, Goldenseal
inflammation	Celery, Chamomile, Chickweed, Devil's claw, Goldenseal, Gotu kola, Oatstraw, Pygeum, Sage, Turmeric, White oak
insomnia	Ashwaganda, Chamomile, Hops, Kava-kava, Lemon balm, Passionflower, Skullcap, Valerian
liver disorders	Milk thistle, Schisandra, Turmeric
low blood pressure	Broom
memory loss, age-related	Ginkgo

menopausal difficulties	Black cohosh, Dong-quai, Red clover, Vitex
menstrual difficulties	Black cohosh, Blue cohosh, Dong-quai, Motherwort, Parsley, Vitex
migraine headaches	Feverfew
motion sickness	Ginger
mouth and throat inflammation	Calendula, Neem
nausea	Chamomile, Ginger, Peppermint
pain relief	Arnica, Devil's claw
PMS	Black cohosh, Dong-quai, Evening primrose, Vitex
sore throat	Bilberry, Calendula, Marshmallow, Slippery elm
stimulant, mild	Damiana
stress	Ashwaganda, Kava-kava
tendency to bruising	Bilberry
tinnitus	Ginkgo
ulcers, stomach or duodenal	Licorice
urinary tract infections, mild	Bearberry, Cranberry
varicose veins	Bilberry, Grapeseed, Horse chestnut

Alfalfa

Medicago sativa

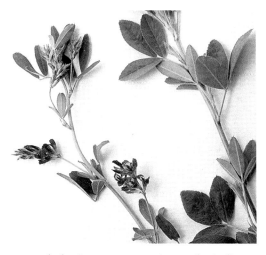

Source: Alfalfa is the dried leaf of a well-known pea family member, with purple flowers and clover-like leaves. It is native to western Asia and the eastern Mediterranean region and is widely grown as fodder for farm animals.

Traditional Use: Alfalfa leaf has been used in tea and dietary supplements to help increase appetite and vitality, reduce water retention, and stimulate digestion and bowel action. It is a folk treatment for rheumatoid arthritis, diabetes, and lowering cholesterol. Its use for loss of energy due to indigestion, dyspepsia, anemia, poor appetite, and weak assimilation began in the early 1900s with American physicians who specialized in herbal medicine. Dr. Ben A. Bradley of Hamlet, Ohio, wrote in 1915: "I find in Alfalfa, after about seven years' clinical tests in my practice and on myself, a superlative restorative tonic. . . . It rejuvenates the whole system by increasing the strength, vim, vigor, and vitality of the patient."

Current Use: Alfalfa has been thoroughly studied as an animal feed but not as an herbal medicine for humans. Animal studies suggest it can prevent high cholesterol in animals on high-fat diets. Compounds in the plant may decrease intestinal absorption of cholesterol and reduce atherosclerotic plaque. Alfalfa is high in protein and contains vitamins A, B1, B6, B12, C, E, and K1, along with the minerals calcium, potassium, phosphorus, iron, and zinc. Despite its widespread use as a dietary supplement, there are no human studies of its claimed benefits. Alfalfa is a good subject for further research.

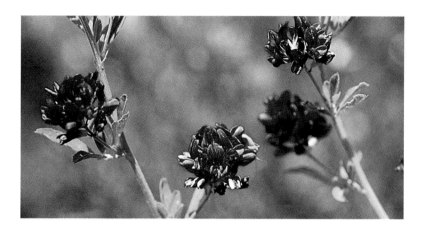

Used For:
Appetite stimulation • Nutrition

Preparations: Dried leaf, capsules, extracts, tablets, tinctures, teas, and others.

Typical Dosages:
Capsules: Up to eight or nine 400–500 mg capsules a day.
Tincture: 15–30 drops 4 times a day.
Or follow manufacturer's or practitioner's recommendations. No therapeutic dosage has been established.

Cautions:
Moderate use of alfalfa products produces no known side effects. One case of allergic reaction (from contamination with grass pollen) in alfalfa tablets has been reported. Eating alfalfa seeds or sprouts has been linked to systemic lupus erythematosus (SLE), a condition characterized by inflammation of connective tissue. In two instances, alfalfa sprouts caused the recurrence of SLE in individuals who had been treated for the condition. Those diagnosed with SLE should avoid alfalfa products. Consuming large quantities of the seeds has also produced reversible blood abnormalities. The compound responsible for ill effects is canavanine.

Aloe Vera

Aloe vera (formerly *A. barbadensis*)

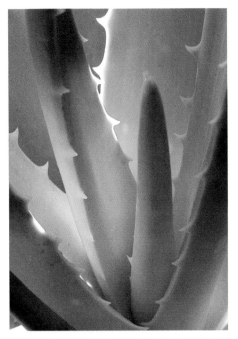

Source: If any herb claims to be America's number-one folk remedy, it is aloe, a succulent perennial of the lily family native to Africa and grown commercially in southern Texas and Mexico. The leaf contains a gooey gel used in medicines and cosmetics; the outer leaf tissue produces a bitter yellow juice, known as drug aloe, once a widely used laxative. Aloe gel should not be confused with drug aloe.

Traditional Use: Aloe gel has been used to treat inflammation for more than 2,500 years. The fresh gel is widely used as a folk medicine for minor burns and sunburn, as well as minor cuts and scrapes. Mixed with water, citric acid, fruit juices, and preservatives, aloe gel is also marketed as "aloe juice," touted as a digestive aid or folk remedy for arthritis, stomach ulcers, diabetes, and other conditions.

Current Use: Modern clinical use of aloe gel began in the 1930s, and recent studies show that aloe gel promotes healing of wounds and burns. Aloe gel relieves pain and inflammation and increases blood supply to injuries by dilating capillaries. It promotes recovery by increasing tensile strength at the wound and healing activity in the space between cells. Recent studies show that topically applied aloe gel significantly increases overall healing rates. A 1995 clinical study by Thai researchers showed that aloe juice held promise for treating new cases of diabetes. In another recent study, a tablespoon of *Aloe vera* juice twice a day reduced triglyceride and blood sugar levels significantly. More research is needed.

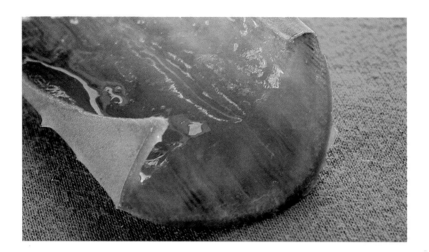

Used For:
First-degree burns • Cuts and abrasions • Wound healing

Preparations:
Gel: Sunscreens, skin creams, lotions, other cosmetics.
Juice: Available in various concentrations and as powdered dry juice. Highly concentrated products degrade quickly; check for inclusion of gums, sugars, starches, and other additives.

Typical Dosages:
Fresh gel: Cut a leaf lengthwise, scrape out the gel, and apply externally as needed. Discontinue if burning or irritation occurs.
Juice: Take 1 tsp after meals, or follow manufacturer's or practitioner's recommendations.

Cautions:
The topical use of aloe gel or aloe-gel products does not usually produce adverse reactions or side effects. There are reports of skin burn following dermal abrasion for removal of acne scars. Rare instances of contact dermatitis (rash) have also been reported. Taking more than the recommended dose of aloe juice may produce a laxative effect.

Arnica

Arnica montana and other species

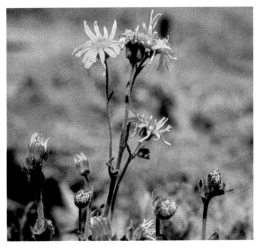

Source: *Arnica* is a genus in the aster family with 32 species in northern temperate regions. The vast majority of arnica species—at least 27—occur in the mountains of western North America. *Arnica montana,* native to Europe, is the primary species used, either the whole plant or, most often, the flowers.

Traditional Use: Preparations of arnica flowers have long been a popular folk remedy, used externally in the form of creams, ointments, or tinctures for the treatment of sprains, bruises, and wound-healing once the wound is closed. Arnica is seldom used internally because of potential toxicity.

> It's Europe's number-one herbal first-aid cream, with as many as 300 products available in the German market alone.

Current Use: Often associated with homeopathic topical products, arnica is widely used externally in Europe as an antiphlogistic, anti-inflammatory, mild pain reliever, and antiseptic for injuries, sprains, bruising, swelling related to bone fractures, insect bites, rheumatic pains, arthralgia, and occasionally phlebitis. In short, it's Europe's number-one herbal first-aid cream, with as many as 300 products available in the German market alone.

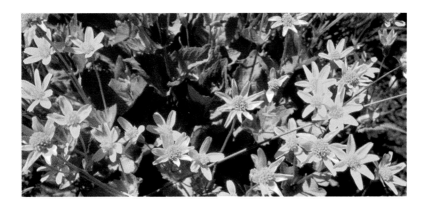

Used For:
Injuries • Pain relief • Reducing inflammation and swelling

Preparations:
Dried flowers, whole or cut and sifted; creams, gels, ointments, tinctures, homeopathic products.

Typical Dosages:
Salves and ointments: Apply externally, follow manufacturer's instructions. It's best to use commercial preparations rather than homemade ones because of arnica's potential toxicity.

Tincture: Internal use of arnica should be done under the guidance of a trained practitioner.

Cautions:
Arnica products should be used only on a short-term basis for acute conditions. They should not be used on damaged, opened, or cracked skin, except under the advice of a health-care practitioner. Continued use can lead to the development of skin pustules or produce an eczema-like reaction. The primary-activity components are considered toxic, so internal use should be avoided (except under medical supervision). Internally, low doses of arnica can cause gastroenteritis; high doses may damage the heart or, in rare cases, lead to cardiac arrest.

Ashwaganda

Withania somnifera

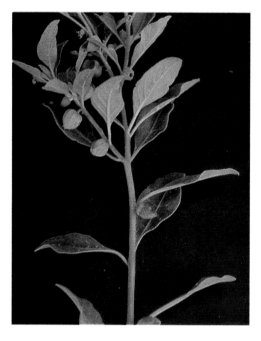

Sources: *Withania somnifera,* a member of the nightshade family native to India, is commonly known as ashwaganda in that country's herbal tradition and as a dietary supplement in the American market. The root of this bushy perennial is used. The supply comes from India, though cultivation of the herb has begun in the United States.

Traditional Use: In Indian traditions ashwaganda has been used as a sedative (hence the species name, *somnifera*). It has been used as a folk medicine as well as an official herb in Ayurvedic medicine, the oldest medical system in the world. It is also official in the *Indian Pharmacopoeia.* In India the use of the herb dates back to Ayurvedic texts at least 3,000 years old. In 100 B.C., a famous physician, Charaka, prescribed it for female disorders and hiccups. For the past 2,000 years, it has been well known in the folk medicine of India as a rejuvenating tonic and aphrodisiac.

Current Use: Interest arose in India during the mid 1950s, when ashwaganda's traditional use as a sedative was first investigated. In India, it is prescribed by physicians as a mild sedative for all types of nervous disorders, including hypertension, and as a treatment for inflammatory joint conditions such as arthritis. Its use in India has been compared to the use of ginseng in China. A recent comparative pharmacological study of ashwaganda and ginseng showed that ashwaganda stimulated the appetite and had significant anabolic activity. It was found to have comparable antistress activity compared with ginseng. The active compounds have been deemed withanolides. Various studies in India have suggested that the herb has significant antioxidant activity, and is an aphrodisiac, anti-inflammatory, and sedative. Since most of this research has been published in scientific journals not available in the United States, the herb has remained somewhat obscure to both the scientific community and mainstream consumers.

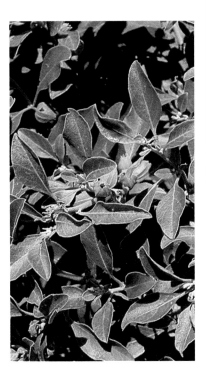

Used For:
Insomnia • Stress

Preparations:
Dried root, powdered; standardized extracts, tinctures.

Typical Dosage:
No therapeutic dosage has been established. For purchased products, follow the manufacturer's or practitioner's recommendations.

Cautions:
Toxicity is generally not associated with the ingestion of small amounts of ashwaganda root. The berries have reportedly caused severe gastroenteritis in children.

Astragalus

Astragalus membranaceus

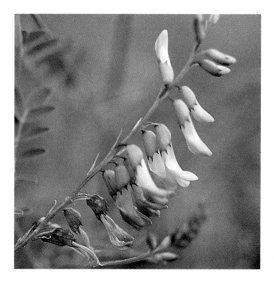

Sources: Astragalus is the root of *Astragalus membranaceus* or *A. membranaceus* var. *mongholicus* (*A. mongholicus*), members of the pea family native to northeast China, where astragalus is commercially grown. Cultivation has also begun in the United States. In China, the root is called *huang-qi*.

Traditional Use: Astragalus is first mentioned in the 2,000-year-old classic, *Shen Nong Ben Cao Jing*. The Chinese name *huang-qi* means "yellow leader"; it is one of the superior tonic roots in Traditional Chinese Medicine. It has been used to invigorate vital energy (Qi) and in prescriptions for shortness of breath, general weakness, and lack of appetite; it has also been used as a diuretic, and for the treatment of colds, flu, stomach ulcers, and diabetes. It is widely used in modern herbal practice in China.

Current Use: Numerous studies by Asian scientists confirm the immunostimulant, antibacterial, antiviral, anti-inflammatory, adaptogenic, and diuretic effects of astragalus. It also improves stamina. No single compound is responsible for its wide-ranging effects, though polysaccharides are involved in immunostimulant activity.

Since 1975, astragalus has been used in China in cancer patients undergoing radiation treatment and chemotherapy. Conventional cancer treatments reduce the function of the immune system; astragalus helps return it to normal. The herb's positive effects on the cardiovascular system have also been extensively studied in China.

In a study done in the early 1980s, researchers in Houston, Texas, found that a chemical fraction extract of astragalus restored T-cell function in seventeen of nineteen cancer patients. In laboratory experiments, water extracts of astragalus root have been found to have an antimutagenic effect, suggesting chemopreventative activity. While astragalus has also been found to have antiviral activity in a number of animal test models, studies on the use of the extract against HIV virus have proved negative.

Used For:
Colds • Flu • Minor infections

Preparations:
Dried root, sliced (looks like a tongue depressor), or powdered; capsules, extracts, tablets, tinctures, combination products.

Typical Dosages:
Capsules: Eight or nine 400–500 mg capsules daily.
Tincture: 15–30 drops 2 times a day.
Or follow manufacturer's or practitioner's recommendations.

Cautions:
No side effects or adverse reactions have been reported.

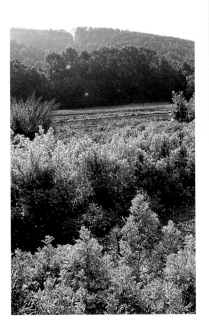

Bearberry

Arctostaphylos uva-ursi

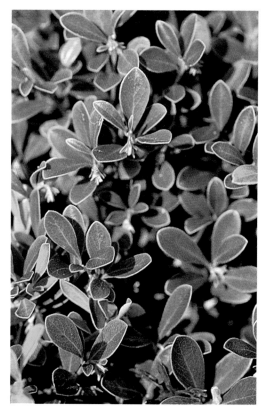

Source: Bearberry, or uva-ursi, is the leaf of a member of the heath family. This trailing, low-growing evergreen shrub is found in cool temperate regions of the Northern Hemisphere, including North America, Europe, and Asia. Most of the leaf in commerce is wild harvested.

Traditional Use: Bearberry's astringent leaves have been used for diarrhea, dysentery, bladder infections, and other afflictions of the urinary tract. Folk medicine has used the herb to treat bronchitis. Long used as a urinary antiseptic by physicians, bearberry was official in the *United States Pharmacopoeia* from 1820 to 1926.

Bearberry was official in the *United States Pharmacopoeia* from 1820 to 1926.

Current Use: Bearberry is an example of an herb whose safe and effective use is far more complicated than simply preparing a tea. While often described as a "diuretic," bearberry does not strongly promote urination but rather serves as a urinary antiseptic if the urine is alkaline. It contains arbutin and methylarbutin which are transformed into hydroquinone in the intestine. A string of chemical reactions results in the inhibition or death of bacteria in the urinary tract. In Germany, bearberrry is approved as a urinary antiseptic.

Used For:
Mild urinary tract infections

Preparations:
Dried herb; capsules, tablets, teas, tinctures.

Typical Dosages:
Capsules: Up to nine 400–500 mg capsules a day.
Infusion: Soak 1/3 ounce of dried leaves in a quart of cold water for 24 hours. Remove leaves and simmer liquid down to 1/2 quart. Take 1 to 2 fluid ounces 3 times a day. Bearberry is only effective if the system is alkaline, so take 2 tsp baking soda in a glass of water each day while using the infusion.
Tincture (1:5, 50% alcohol): 30–60 drops in a cup of water 3 times a day.
Or follow manufacturer's or practitioner's recommendations.

Cautions:
Bearberry is high in tannins, which can produce stomachache, nausea, and vomiting. If you have a weak stomach, avoid bearberry. It is generally not recommended for children. Use should not be continued for more than a week except under the direction of a health-care practitioner, as overuse may cause liver damage. If you suspect you have a kidney disorder, consult your health-care practitioner. Kidney disease cannot be self-diagnosed and should not be self-treated. Avoid bearberry during pregnancy.

Bilberry
Vaccinium myrtillus

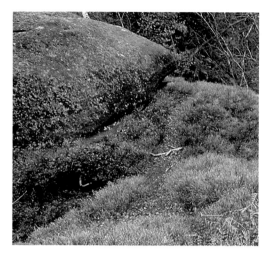

Source: Bilberry, a relative of blueberry and bearberry, belongs to the heath family. A small shrub with sweet black berries, it grows in the heaths and woods of northern Europe, as well as in western Asia and the Rocky Mountains. The berries and leaves are used.

Traditional Use: An ancient food plant of Europe, bilberry emerged as a medicinal herb in the sixteenth century. The leaves were used for their astringent, tonic, anti-inflammatory, and antiseptic qualities.

Tea made from the dried berries was used as an astringent for diarrhea and dysentery, a diuretic, and a cooling nutritive tonic. It was also used to prevent scurvy (vitamin C deficiency), to stop bleeding, and as a disinfectant for mouth inflammations.

During World War II, pilots in the British Royal Air Force reported improved night vision after eating bilberry jam. In the 1960s, these reports led Italian and French scientists to research the berries for their effects on vision problems.

Current Use: In Europe, preparations of bilberry fruit are used to enhance poor microcirculation, thus improving eye conditions such as night blindness and diabetic

> **During World War II, pilots in the British Royal Air Force reported improved night vision after eating bilberry jam.**

retinopathy. Pigments called anthocyanosides help regenerate a pigment in the retina that is essential for the eye to adapt to light.

Fragile capillaries, a common condition in the elderly, can result in easy bruising, poor blood circulation to connective tissues, and inflammatory conditions such as arthritis. Anthocyanosides in bilberry strengthen capillaries by protecting them from free radical damage. They also stimulate the formation of healthy connective tissue. Bilberry may reduce blood platelet stickiness (platelet aggregation), a risk factor associated with atherosclerosis. Bilberry is recommended for managing varicose veins and hemorrhoids, and rebuilding healthy connective tissue, but unfortunately most studies have involved animals or only a small number of humans. In Germany, the dried berries are sold for treating mild diarrhea and minor inflammations of the mucous membranes of the throat and mouth.

Used For:
Atherosclerosis • Bruising • Diarrhea • Hemorrhoids • Microcirculation • Mouth and throat inflammation • Tendency to bruising • Varicose veins

Preparations:
Dried fruit; capsules, tablets. Standardized products contain 25% anthocyanosides.

Typical Dosage:
Capsules and tablets: 2 or 3 standardized capsules or tablets a day. Or follow manufacturer's or practitioner's recommendations.

Cautions:
No side effects, contraindications, or interactions with other drugs have been reported.

Black Cohosh

Cimicifuga racemosa

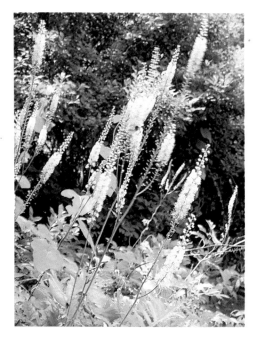

Source: Black cohosh, the root of a member of the buttercup family, is found in rich woods of the eastern deciduous forests from southern Ontario south to Georgia, west to Arkansas, and north to Wisconsin. Most of the root is wild harvested, while some is grown commercially in Europe.

Traditional Use: Among Native Americans and early North American settlers, black cohosh root was an important folk medicine for menstrual irregularities and childbirth. Adopted in medical practice in the early nineteenth century, it had a great reputation for both these purposes and as an anti-inflammatory for arthritis and rheumatism. It was also used for nervous disorders. The root was an official drug in the *U. S. Pharmacopoeia* from 1820 to 1926.

Current Use: Black cohosh is approved for use in Germany for the treatment of premenstrual symptoms, painful or difficult menstruation, and for menopausal symptoms such as hot flashes. A number of studies have confirmed its mild sedative and anti-inflammatory activity. An isoflavone in the root binds to estrogen receptors, producing estrogen-like activity. As ovarian function declines during menopause, estrogen production also declines and luteinizing hormone (LH) increases. These changes are associated with hot flashes. In one study an alcohol extract of black cohosh reduced hot flashes in animals and women by lowering LH.

Another study compared the effects of conventional estrogen replacement therapy with black cohosh in sixty women less than forty years old who had had complete hysterectomies and were experiencing abrupt menopause. In all groups, LH reduction indicates that treatment with black cohosh compares to conventional treatment.

Black cohosh has been widely used in Europe for over forty years, with documentation in over 1.5 million cases. Efficacy and safety are confirmed by this long-term clinical experience, as well as recent controlled clinical studies.

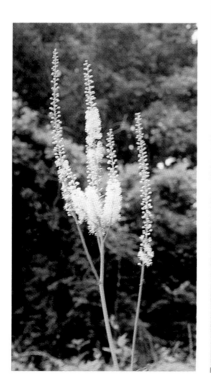

Used For:
Menstrual difficulties • Menopausal difficulties • PMS

Preparations:
Dried root; capsules, tablets, tinctures. Standardized products are available.

Typical Dosage:
Capsules: Three 500–600 mg capsules a day of the whole herb.
Tincture (1:5, 80% alcohol): 10–25 drops as often as every 4 hours.
Or follow manufacturer's or practitioner's recommendations.

Cautions:
No contraindications or drug interactions are reported, though some women have experienced upset stomach from use of black cohosh preparations. A long term toxicity study in animals showed no adverse effects.

Blessed Thistle

Centaurea benedictus (formerly *Cnicus benedictus*)

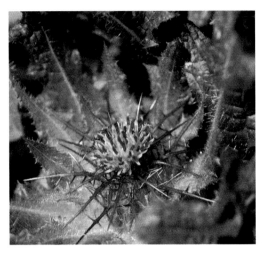

Sources: The above-ground part of the plant is harvested in flower. A member of the aster family, blessed thistle is a weed of the fields and waste places in the Mediterranean region and is cultivated elsewhere in herb gardens. It has escaped and established itself sporadically in the United States and Canada. While botanists currently classify it as *Centaurea benedictus,* virtually all herb books refer to it under the long-established name *Cnicus benedictus.*

Traditional Use: Also known as holy thistle (but not to be confused with milk thistle, *Silybum marianum*), the whole herb has been used to promote digestion, induce sweating, and regulate the menses. Culpepper and other early herbalists listed blessed thistle as a remedy for stomach complaints, liver problems, and to stimulate bile secretion. Externally it was used for everything from bites of rabid dogs to treating sores caused by bubonic plague. It is still used topically to stop bleeding from wounds and, in British herbal traditions, to treat sores.

> **Externally it was used for everything from bites of rabid dogs to treating sores caused by bubonic plague.**

Current Use: The herb is still official in the pharmacopoeias of Austria and Hungary. The primary use is as a bitter tonic to stimulate digestion in cases of dyspepsia or stomach upset accompanied by gas. Various components have been found to possess activity against a wide range of bacteria. The primary action of the herb is to increase the appetite by stimulating secretion of gastric juice and saliva. While human studies are absent from the literature, pharmacological studies confirm traditional use as a bitter digestive tonic, as an antibacterial agent, and as an anti-inflammatory.

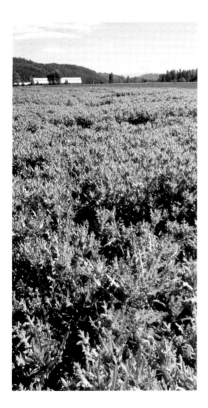

Used For:
Digestion • Stimulating appetite

Preparations:
Dried herb, cut and sifted; capsules, tablets, tonics, and tinctures.

Typical Dosages:
Capsules: Three 500–600 mg capsules a day.
Tea: Steep 1–2 tsp cut and sifted dried herb in a cup of hot water for 10–15 minutes. Use up to 3 times a day a half-hour before meals.
Or follow manufacturer's or practitioner's recommendations.

Cautions:
Those with allergic reactions to aster family plants should avoid using the herb. Extremely rare allergic reactions are possible, including contact dermatitis.

Blue Cohosh

Caulophyllum thalictroides

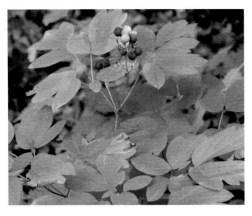

Sources: Blue cohosh is the rhizome (underground stem) of a member of the barberry family found in rich woodlands of eastern North America. It occurs from New Brunswick and Ontario south to South Carolina, Alabama, and the Ozarks. Two North American species are now recognized, *C. thalictroides* and *C. giganteum*. The two are not distinguished in the herb trade. A third species, *C. robustum*, is found in Japan.

Traditional Use: Long used by Native Americans as a childbirth aid, blue cohosh became known to the medical community through an 1813 publication by a self-styled "Indian herb doctor," Peter Smith. Indian women are said to have employed a decoction of the root, drunk two or three weeks before childbirth, to help facilitate delivery. In nineteenth-century medical practice, it was used to reduce muscle spasms, treat menstrual disorders, induce sweating, and as a diuretic. The rhizome of the Asian species *C. robustum* has been used in folk traditions to treat menstrual disorders, stomach problems, injuries from fractures, and rheumatism.

> **Indian women are said to have employed a decoction of the root, drunk two or three weeks before childbirth, to help facilitate delivery.**

Current Use: Modern herbalists recommend blue cohosh to stimulate the uterus, promote menstruation, and reduce spasms. Under the care of an experienced midwife familiar with the herb's specific actions, it is most often used to help pass the placenta. A rat study has shown that an extract inhibits ovulation and implantation, suggesting potential for contraceptive research. Scientific studies have found an alkaloid, methylcytisine, which increases blood pressure, stimulates respiration, and aids the function of the small intestine in much the same way as nicotine. Traditional use coupled with current research sets the foundation for the need of further research on this active herb.

Used For:
Menstrual disturbances

Preparations:
Dried root, cut and sifted; capsules, tablets, tinctures, combination products.

Typical Dosage:
Tincture (1:5, 60% alcohol): 5–20 drops up to 4 times a day.
Or follow manufacturer's or practitioner's recommendations.

Cautions:
There is no doubt that blue cohosh is a powerful herb, its use best supervised by knowledgeable practitioners. It should be avoided during pregnancy except under medical advice. Generally it is used by practitioners only after labor has begun. This herb should be used with caution.

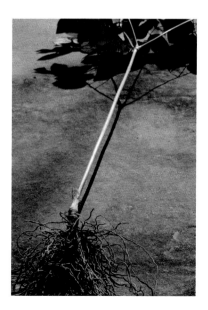

Boldo

Peumus boldo

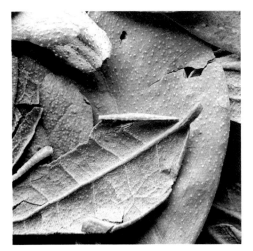

Sources: Boldo is the dried leaves of a member of the monimia family, found in the Andes of Argentina, Bolivia, Chile, Ecuador, and Peru. It is an evergreen shrub growing to 25-feet in height with smooth, leathery leaves.

Traditional Use: In South America, boldo is used not only as a medicinal tea, but as a spice. One European observer of the early eighteenth century found that the Indians of Chile used the leaves to control gout. Various South American folk traditions use boldo tea for liver, bladder, and prostate ailments, to expel gas from the intestines, stimulate digestion, and reduce fever. The medical profession was introduced to the herb by a French physician in 1872. Papers delivered before pharmaceutical societies in Great Britain and Philadelphia in 1875 brought its medicinal value to wider attention. It was used in the late nineteenth century for gastric pain, nervous conditions, jaundice, dyspepsia, liver conditions, and as a diuretic.

> **In South America, boldo is used not only as a medicinal tea, but as a spice.**

Current Use: In modern European herbal medicine, boldo leaves are used to treat mild digestive disturbances and stimulate release of bile into the intestines. Boldo contains an essential oil responsible for its aroma, but the primary active constituent is the alkaloid boldine. Various laboratory studies on extracts of the leaves, as well as pure boldine, have found that boldo can help protect the liver against toxic compounds, that it has a smooth-muscle relaxant effect and antioxidant activity. A recent limited clinical study on twelve patients shows that boldo prolongs intestinal transit time. German health authorities allow its use for mild gastrointestinal upset accompanied by cramps and dyspeptic complaints.

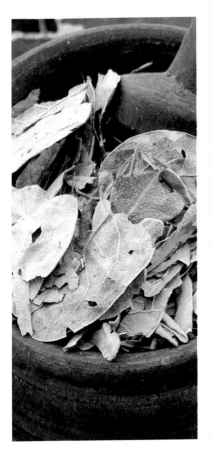

Used For:
Diuresis • Gastric spasms • Bile release

Preparations:
Dried leaves, whole or ground; capsules, tablets, tinctures, and other preparations. Often combined with other products in weight-loss formulations.

Typical Dosage:
Tea: Steep 1–2 tsp dried, ground herb in 1 cup hot water for 10–15 minutes. Use once a day.
Or follow manufacturer's or practitioner's recommendations.

Cautions: According to European authorities, boldo should be avoided in cases of liver or gallbladder obstruction and used under a physician's supervision for gallstones. Use should be limited to one month; avoid use during pregnancy and lactation. No side effects are generally reported. However, the essential oil contains toxic components and should be avoided.

Borage

Borago officinalis

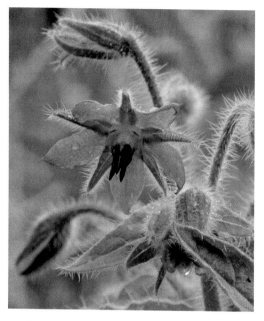

Sources: Borage (*Borago officinalis*) is a common annual European herb, widely grown in herb gardens. Historically, the leaves of borage were used as a folk medicine. The flowers are a delicate addition to salads. Most modern interest is in the seed oil, a source of gamma-linolenic acid.

Traditional Use: In the first century both Pliny the Elder and Dioscorides identified borage as Homer's famous "nepenthe" which, when steeped in wine, produced "absolute forgetfulness." In medieval times borage was associated with mirth, courage, and "gladdening the heart." The effect of the leaves was considered cooling and diuretic. The leaf tea was used for fevers, jaundice, and rheumatism, and externally to heal wounds and as an anti-inflammatory. Due to potential toxicity, use of the leaves has waned.

Current Status: Like the oil of evening primrose (which see), the seed oil of borage is a rich source of gamma-linolenic acid, an essential fatty acid, deficient in some individuals, but necessary in the manufacture of key chemical mediators in the body. In short, borage is the richest known plant source of this essential fatty acid. One rat study showed that borage oil may reduce reaction to stress, and a limited chemical study on ten individuals found that borage oil reduces stress by lowering systolic blood pressure and heart rate. Even though borage oil has components similar to those of evening primrose oil, studies of the latter do not apply to borage oil.

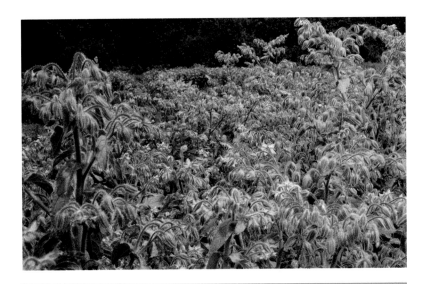

Used For:
Deficiency of essential fatty acids

Preparations:
Capsules containing borage seed oil.

Typical Dosage:
Capsules: Three to four 300 mg capsules a day.
Or follow manufacturer's or practitioner's recommendations.

Cautions:
Like evening primrose oil, borage oil should be used with caution in cases of epilepsy, or by individuals taking phenothiazine drugs. Like comfrey leaves (also in the borage family), borage leaves contain potentially toxic and carcinogenic alkaloids (but in much smaller concentrations than comfrey). The effects of the alkaloids can be cumulative; even minute levels can pose danger. Consumption of the leaves, either fresh or dried, is best avoided.

Broom

Cytisus scoparius

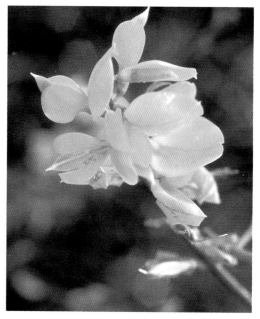

Sources: Broom (*Cytisus scoparius*, syn. *Sarothamnus scoparius*) comes from the leaves of a shrub in the pea family native to Europe and now commonly naturalized in North and South America. In older works it is sometimes found under the name scoparius.

Traditional Use: The leaves of broom were mentioned in the earliest Italian, German, and Anglo-Saxon herbals. John Gerarde in *The Herball* (1597), notes that Henry VII used it "against surfets and disease thereof arising." This European species has been the emblem of several English kings. It has long been used as a diuretic (in small doses). In larger doses, it may produce vomiting, sweating, and impaired vision. The green tender tops were once used to flavor beer.

> **Herbalists use broom to treat poor circulation or heart conditions, especially low blood pressure.**

Current Use: Broom contains a number of alkaloids that are considered responsible for its medicinal effects, especially sparteine (at 0.3 to 0.8 percent). Herbalists use broom to treat poor circulation or heart conditions, especially low blood pressure. In a tea, the herb can help improve circulation. Sparteine, the main alkaloid, has potential to restore normal heart rhythm in arrhythmic patients. The plant has long been used in folk traditions around the world, but is best used today under medical supervision.

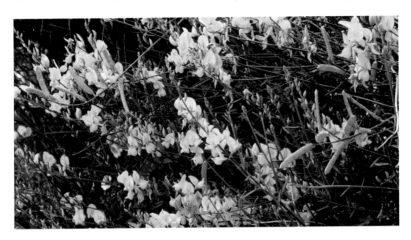

Used For:
Diuretic • Heart arrhythmia • Low blood pressure

Preparations:
Dried herb, cut and sifted; capsules, tablets, tinctures, other liquid extract forms.

Typical Dosages:
Tea: Steep 1/2–1 tsp dried herb in 1 cup hot water for 10–15 minutes.
Tincture: 20–30 drops a day.
Or follow manufacturer's or practitioner's recommendations.

Cautions:
As with any heart-affecting preparation, broom should be used with caution. It should not be used in cases of high blood pressure or hypertension. If heart disease is present, use under the supervision of a physician. Avoid use during pregnancy and lactation.

Burdock

Arctium lappa, A. minus

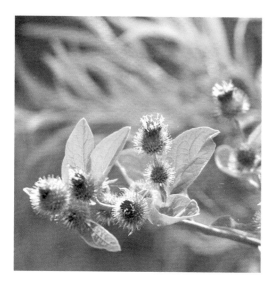

Sources: The roots, leaves, and seeds of burdock, a common weed in the aster family, have all been used as sources of herbal products. Burdock is an Old World temperate-climate species that occurs throughout much of the northern hemisphere. In Japan, it is commonly grown as a vegetable for its edible roots, as carrots are in the United States.

Traditional Use: Western herbal traditions mainly use the root as a blood purifier to treat skin conditions such as eczema, psoriasis, and hives. Considered diuretic and slightly laxative, it has been used to disperse kidney stones and treat liver conditions. Externally, a wash of the root has been used to treat slow-to-heal wounds. Although weaker, the leaves have also been used for similar purposes. In Scandinavia, the young leaves are eaten in spring salads. In Traditional Chinese Medicine, the seeds (fruits), known as *niu-bang-zi,* are the main plant part used; in the Western world, the seeds have been used to detoxify the blood, reduce swelling, and clear skin eruptions. Burdock tea has also been used to treat cough, swelling, infections, and other conditions.

Current Use: Little modern research has been conducted on burdock. Root extracts have been shown to produce mild antibiotic activity and to stimulate bile flow from the liver. In animal models, the roots and leaves have been shown to lower blood sugar and increase carbohydrate tolerance.

A number of isolated chemical components from the root, including polyacetylene compounds and a bitter component, arctiopicrin, possess antibacterial action. Several studies have shown that burdock root reduces mutagenic action and protects against the toxicity of artificial food colorings. Antitumor activity has also been observed in animal studies. While chemical and pharmacological studies suggest a rational scientific basis for traditional use, human clinical studies have not been conducted. Use is not approved in Germany because of lack of scientific substantiation of traditional claims.

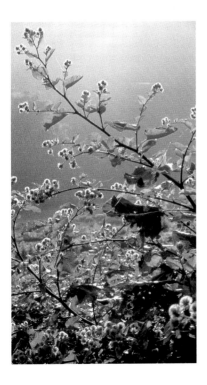

Used For:
Diuresis • Detoxification

Preparations:
Dried root (or leaves), whole or cut and sifted; capsules, liquid extract, tablets, tinctures.

Typical Dosages:
Capsules: Up to six 400–500 mg capsules a day.
Tea: Steep 1 tsp dried root in a cup of hot water for 10–15 minutes. Use up to three times a day.
Tincture (1:5, 50% alcohol): 10–25 drops 3 times a day.
Or follow manufacturer's or practitioner's recommendations.

Cautions:
Generally, no side effects are reported for burdock. One case of human poisoning attributed to burdock is thought to result from contamination or misidentification with highly toxic belladonna leaf.

Calendula

Calendula officinalis

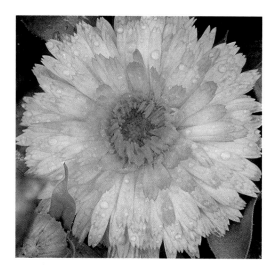

Source: Also known as pot marigold (not to be confused with the common garden marigolds of the *Tagetes* species), calendula is the dried flower of a member of the aster family native to south-central Europe and northern Africa. A garden annual, it is commonly grown for its bright display of yellow or orange flowers.

Traditional Use: The flowers have been applied to cuts and wounds, burns and bruises, and used as a tea for gastric ulcers and other stomach ailments, for jaundice and other conditions.

> **Calendula preparations are approved in Germany and other European countries for topical use on slow-to-heal wounds.**

Current Use: Calendula preparations are approved in Germany and other European countries for topical use on slow-to-heal wounds and for ulcerations on the leg. A gargle or tea is used to reduce inflammation of the mouth or sore throat. Most human studies of the plant have been conducted in eastern European countries and have involved only small numbers of patients. They indicate that extracts of the herb may be of use in treating duodenal ulcers and helping surgical wounds heal.

Pharmacological studies, most involving animals, have confirmed a wide range of activities. Calendula extracts are anti-inflammatory, antiviral, and stimulate the immune system to increase effectiveness of white blood cells. (In this respect, calendula is similar to echinacea.) In addition, calendula increases granulation at the site of a wound, helping grow new healthy cells and increasing the number of micro blood vessels. Topical calendula preparations are widely accepted in Europe for treating inflammation of the skin and mucous membranes, slow-to-heal wounds, mild burns, and sunburn.

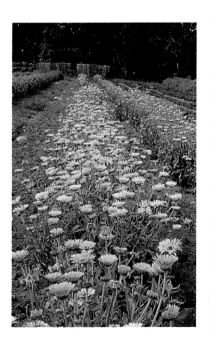

Used For:
First-degree burns • Mouth and throat infections • Sore throat • Wound healing

Preparations:
Dried flowers; salves, tinctures.

Typical Dosages:
Tea: Steep 1 heaping tsp dried flowers in a cup of hot water for 10–15 minutes. Take 3 times a day.
Tincture (1:5, 70% alcohol): 5–40 drops 3 times a day. For external use, apply tincture to affected area.
Or follow manufacturer's or practitioner's recommendations.

Cautions:
Generally no side effects or contraindications have been reported. Persons allergic to the pollen of other members of the aster family, such as ragweed, may also be allergic to calendula. One case of a severe allergic reaction to the tea was reported in Russia.

Cascara Sagrada

Rhamnus purshiana

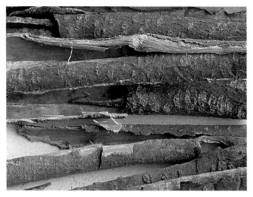

Source: Cascara sagrada is the dried, aged bark of a small tree in the buckthorn family native to the Pacific Northwest. The bark is harvested mostly from wild trees in Oregon, Washington, and southern British Columbia. The bark is aged for a year so that the active principles become milder. Freshly dried bark produces too strong a laxative for safe use; it also contains a compound that induces vomiting.

Traditional Use: Cascara sagrada is Spanish for "sacred bark." Long used as a laxative by Native American groups of the northwest Pacific coast, the bark was not introduced into formal medical practice in the United States until 1877. In 1890, it replaced the berries of the European buckthorn (*R. catharticus*) as an official laxative. Cascara sagrada is still used in over-the-counter laxatives available in pharmacies throughout the United States.

> **Dried, aged cascara sagrada bark is widely accepted as a mild and effective treatment for chronic constipation.**

Current Use: Dried, aged cascara sagrada bark is widely accepted as a mild and effective treatment for chronic constipation. The bark contains compounds called anthraquinones (cascarosides A and B) which are transformed by intestinal bacteria into substances that increase peristalsis in the large intestine and help restore its tone.

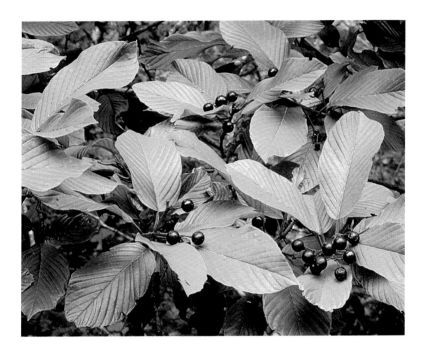

Used For:
Constipation

Preparations:
Dried bark (very bitter); capsules, extracts.

Typical Dosages:
Capsules: Up to two 400–500 mg capsules a day.
Liquid extract: 1/2 to 1 teaspoon.
Or follow manufacturer's or practitioner's recommendations.

Cautions:
Only use aged bark. If you have chronic constipation, see your doctor for other approaches to avoid laxative dependency.

Cat's-Claw

Uncaria tomentosa, U. guianensis

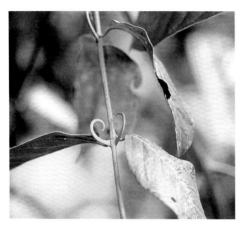

Sources: Cat's-claw (*una de gato*) comes from the stem and root of two Amazonian woody vines belonging to the madder family. Both species are used interchangeably in South America. Commercial supplies are wild-harvested in Peru and Brazil.

Traditional Use: The Piura Indians used a bark decoction of *U. guianensis* to treat inflammation, rheumatism, gastric ulcers, and tumors, and as a contraceptive. Today *U. tomentosa* is a South American folk medicine for intestinal ailments, gastric ulcers, dysentery, arthritis, wounds, and cancer. Popular use in North America started in the 1990s.

Current Use: Reports of successful use as a South American folk remedy for cancer have prompted scientists in Germany, Austria, and Italy to take a closer look at cat's-claw. In the 1970s compounds called proanthocyanidins were found to inhibit tumor growth in animals. Studies at the University of Munich in 1985 found several alkaloids in cat's-claw root with significant immunostimulant activity. In 1993, preliminary pharmacological tests in Italy found new compounds that show antiviral, antimutagenic, and antioxidant effects. An Austrian research group has found several alkaloids that inhibit the growth of tumor cells in laboratory tests. Cat's-claw root may be as much as four times stronger than stem bark.

In Germany and Austria, physicians have given standardized cat's-claw extracts to cancer patients to stimulate their immune system. Extracts have also been used in cases of rheumatoid arthritis, allergies, herpes infections, gastric ulcers, gastritis, and AIDS. Cat's-claw products are registered pharmaceuticals in Germany and Austria and are available only by prescription.

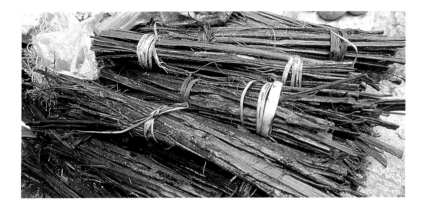

Used For:
Inflammation • Stimulating immunity

Preparations:
Dried root and stem, cut and sifted or powdered; capsules, extracts, tablets, tinctures. Products standardized for total alkaloid content are available.

Typical Dosages:
Capsules: Up to nine 500–600 mg capsules a day.
Decoction: Simmer 1 tbsp pulverized root in 1 qt water for 45 minutes. Take 1 tsp in hot water before breakfast.
Tincture: 20–40 drops up to 5 times a day.
Or follow manufacturer's or practitioner's recommendations.

Cautions:
Like other immunostimulants, cat's-claw should be avoided in diseases of the immune system itself, such as tuberculosis, multiple sclerosis, and HIV infection. It is not known to be safe for children or pregnant or nursing women. In Germany and Austria, therapies using cat's-claw standardized products are not allowed to be combined with therapies involving hormones, insulin, fresh blood plasma, vaccines, or in certain other special situations. Consult a physician before using cat's-claw.

Cayenne

Capsicum annuum, C. frutescens

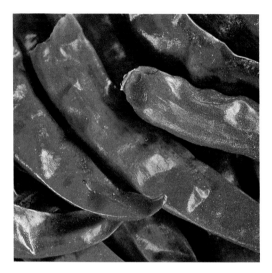

Source: Cayenne is the pungent dried fruit of a highly variable species in the nightshade family that also produces paprika, bell, and jalapeño peppers. Cayenne originates in the tropical Americas and is grown worldwide.

Traditional Use: The ancient Maya used cayenne to treat mouth sores and inflamed gums. Herbal use as a stimulant began with Samuel Thomson (1769–1843), who used it to "produce a strong heat in the body" and "restore digestive powers." In the 1970s John Christopher promoted cayenne as a circulatory stimulant, claiming that "it feeds the necessary elements into the cell structure of the arteries, veins and capillaries so that these regain the elasticity of youth again, and the blood pressure adjusts itself to normal."

> **The ancient Maya used cayenne to treat mouth sores and inflamed gums.**

Current Use: The popular belief that cayenne stimulates digestion and circulation has no scientific proof; in Germany, therefore, cayenne products are not permitted to carry such claims. Cayenne does, however, contain carotenoids and vitamins C and E; these antioxidants protect against free radicals, oxygen compounds that can damage cell membranes and disturb metabolic pathways. Consumption of carotenoids is associated with a reduced risk of cancer and enhances the activity of various immune system cells. The carotenoids in cayenne have been shown clinically to improve lifespan in primates.

Capsaicin, the source of cayenne's bite, is used in minute amounts in topical pharmaceutical products to treat pain at the site of an apparently healed infection, for shingles and osteo- and rheumatoid arthritis. (The whole herb itself is not used in this way.)

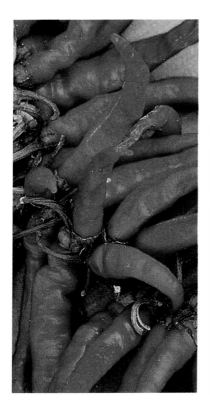

Used For:
Antioxidant action • Nutrition

Preparations:
Fresh or dried powdered fruit; capsules, tablets, tinctures.

Typical Dosages:
Capsules: Up to three 400–500 mg capsules a day.
Spice: Use freely in flavoring food.
Tea: Steep 1/2–1 tsp powdered spice in a cup of hot water for 10–15 minutes.
Tincture: 5–10 drops in water. Or follow manufacturer's or practitioner's recommendations.

Cautions:
Cayenne's pungent principal, capsaicin, is a highly toxic irritant in its pure form. Capsaicin is not water soluble, so it is difficult to wash off after one handles hot peppers. Scientists working with capsaicin protect themselves with space-suit garb. Hot peppers can cause burning skin irritation, a condition called "Hunan hand" from the spicy cuisine of Hunan, China.

Celery

Apium graveolens

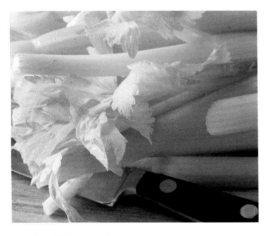

Sources: A stout biennial native to Europe, celery includes varieties grown for seed (fruit), stems, and root (celeriac). Oils from the fruits are used in the manufacturing of processed food. The majority of the world's supply of celery seed and oil comes from India.

Traditional Use: Celery stems and leaves have been used as an aphrodisiac, diuretic, mild sedative to relieve muscle spasms, and anti-inflammatory. Traditionally, celery is best known for treating asthma, bronchitis, gout, and rheumatism, and as a "blood purifier." Celery seeds have been valued as a stimulant and carminative, as well as a mild nerve sedative and tonic.

> **Current interest in celery-seed extracts is driven by folkloric use to reduce uric-acid levels, thereby easing the pain and inflammation of arthritis, rheumatism, and gout.**

Current Use: Current interest in celery-seed extracts is driven by folkloric use to reduce uric-acid levels, thereby easing the pain and inflammation of arthritis, rheumatism, and gout. Medicinal plant expert Dr. James A. Duke has reported personal success with using a celery-seed extract for gout, though clinical studies are currently lacking. Eating celery stalks has also been associated with reduced blood pressure and lowered risk of heart disease.

Celery research has concentrated on the effects of a unique compound, 3-n-butylphthalide, shown to significantly reduce total serum cholesterol levels. The compound displays anti-inflammatory activity, lowers blood sugar, reduces muscle spasms, and lowers the concentration of stress hormones in the blood. Celery whole plant, root, herb, and seed are the subject of a German Commission E monograph. Since effectiveness has not been scientifically proven, no therapeutic claims are allowed.

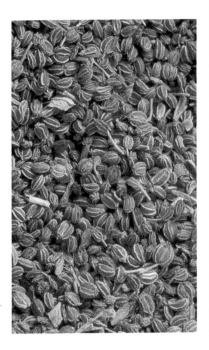

Used For:
Diuresis • Inflammation

Preparations:
Fresh stalks; dried seed, seed extract.

Typical Dosages:
Extract of seed: Follow manufacturer's instructions.
Fresh stalks: Eat 4 or more stalks a day as part of a blood-pressure reduction diet.
Tea: Steep 1/4–1 tsp of seeds in hot water for 10 minutes.

Cautions:
If you have kidney inflammation, avoid celery seed. Some individuals are sensitive to celery, which may cause allergic reactions or contact dermatitis. Individuals sensitive to birch and/or mugwort pollen can have an immediate hypersensitivity to ingesting celery. Celery also contains psoralen, which can cause photodermatitis when the skin is exposed to the sun. In one isolated case, a woman had a severe phototoxic reaction after eating celery root (celeriac), then going to a tanning salon.

Chamomile

Matricaria recutita (formerly *M. chamomilla, Chamomilla recutita*)

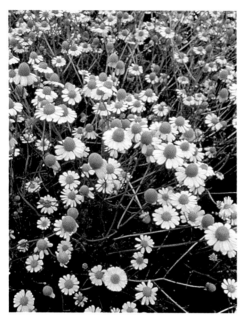

Source: Chamomile (or German camomile) is the dried flower head of an annual member of the aster family. The primary chamomile of commerce, it is grown in Hungary, the Czech Republic, Slovakia, Germany, Argentina, and Egypt. Roman (or English) chamomile, the flower of the perennial *Chamaemelum nobile* (formerly *Anthemis nobilis*), is less frequently seen in the American market.

Traditional Use: According to Varro Tyler, Germans call chamomile *alles zutraut*—"capable of anything." A Slovakian chamomile specialist, Ivan Salamon, states, "Chamomile is the most-favored and most-used medicinal plant in Slovakia. Our folk saying maintains that an individual should always bow when facing a chamomile plant. This respect results from hundreds of years' experience with curing in the folk medicine of the country." Chamomile has been used for centuries to quiet an upset stomach, promote urination and relieve colic, and induce sleep. Topically, chamomile has been used to reduce inflammation, soothe aches, and heal cuts, sores, and bruises.

Current Use: Chamomile is an official drug in the pharmacopoeias of twenty-six countries, and its uses today differ little from those of ancient times. It is used as an anti-inflammatory, antiseptic, carminative, antispasmodic, and mild sedative, as well as for promotion of wound healing. In Europe, chamomile is used externally in compresses, rinses, or gargles; to treat inflammations and irritations of the skin and mucous membranes, including the mouth, gums, and respiratory tract; and for hemorrhoids. Chamomile tea or tincture relieves spasms and inflammation of the gastrointestinal tract as well as peptic ulcers. A mild tea makes a gentle sleep aid, particularly for children. Modern indications are backed not only by intensive recent research (except for sleep-aid claims), but by many centuries of common use.

Used For:
Indigestion • Insomnia • Nausea • Inflammation • Wound healing

Preparations:
Dried flowers; capsules, cream salve, tea, tincture, bath products.

Typical Dosages:
Bath: For hemorrhoids or irritated skin, soak 1 lb of dried flowers in a tub of hot water.
Capsules: Up to six 300–400 mg capsules a day.
Tea: Steep 1/2–1 tsp dried flowers in a cup of hot water. Use 3 to 4 times a day.
Tincture: 10–40 drops 3 times a day.
Or follow manufacturer's or practitioner's recommendations.

Cautions:
Persons allergic to the pollen of other members of the aster family, such as ragweed, may also be allergic to chamomile. Teas made from the dried flowers contain pollen. Chamomile is associated with rare contact dermatitis. At least one case of anaphylactic shock has been attributed to consumption of chamomile tea. Varro Tyler points out, however, that of fifty reported allergic reactions to "chamomiles," only five have been attributed to German chamomile, a figure that attests to the herb's relative safety. Worldwide, approximately a million cups of chamomile tea are consumed daily.

Chaparral

Larrea tridentata

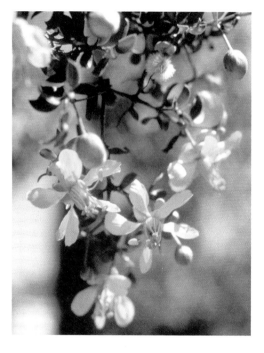

Sources: The herb chaparral consists of the dried, highly resinous leaves of *Larrea tridentata,* a common shrub in the caltrop family found in deserts of North America. A dominant desert flora, chaparral covers thousands of square miles from California, Utah, Arizona, and New Mexico west to Texas and south to Mexico.

Traditional Use: The leaves were used by Native Americans to induce vomiting, treat diarrhea, and ease menstrual cramps. Externally the leaves were used for scratches, sores, wounds, bruises, and to treat rheumatism. In Mormon traditions in Utah, the plant has a reputation as a folk cancer remedy. This use has attracted modern attention to the herb.

Current Use: Major uses of chaparral depend on its antioxidant, anti-inflammatory, antimicrobial, and purported antitumor properties. In 1969, a research group in Salt Lake City became interested in chapparal's anti tumor activity because a patient taking chaparral experienced a remission of a malignant melanoma. A subsequent clinical trial conducted on fifty-nine patients with various types of tumors produced no significant statistical evidence of anticancer activity. However, some tumor regressions were reported. Side effects from the use of chaparral include gastrointestinal symptoms, rash, stomatitis, and fever.

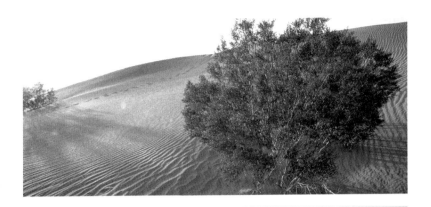

Used For:
Folk cancer remedy

Preparations:
Until the early 1990s, available as dried herb or capsules, tablets, tinctures, and extracts. However it has become increasingly difficult to find in the market (see Cautions).

Typical Dosage:
Older promotional literature suggests about a teaspoon of the dried leaves made into a tea. For commercial products, follow manufacturer's or practitioner's recommendations.

Cautions:
On December 10, 1992, the FDA Center for Food Safety and Applied Nutrition issued a press release warning of the potential link between use of chaparral and liver toxicity. At least four cases of serious liver problems following chaparral use and requiring hospitalization were reported to the Centers for Disease Control. Shortly after that, industry trade associations asked their members to suspend sales of the herb. It remains unknown whether the herb is inherently toxic or if contamination occurred, but regulatory authorities and trade groups still encourage manufacturers not to sell chaparral products.

Chickweed

Stellaria media

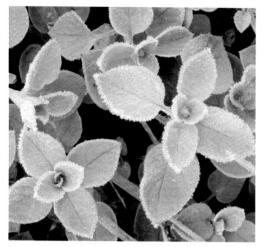

Sources: Chickweed is the whole herb of *S. media,* a member of the pink family, thought to be native to southern Europe, but now a common weed throughout much of the world. Both the fresh and dried herb are used. Most commercial supplies come from eastern Europe.

Traditional Use: In various herbal traditions, chickweed is considered cooling and soothing to irritated mucous membranes. Native Americans washed sore eyes with an infusion of the weed and applied fresh leaves to soothe cuts and sores. British folk traditions have used the fresh leaves as a poultice for carbuncles or abscesses. In teas the dried herb has been used to treat coughs and hoarseness. The fresh leaves, which appear in early spring, are a wild edible that's excellent in salads. Nineteenth-century physicians recommended chickweed tincture for rheumatism.

Current Use: Chickweed is generally absent from major works on scientific aspects of herbal medicine. Compounds from the roots of the Asian *S. dichotoma* var. *lanceolata* and *S. yunnanensis* have been researched for potential anticancer and antioxidant activity. The fresh herb of common chickweed contains appreciable amounts of vitamin C as well as protein. A number of chemical groups, including glycosides, flavonoids, saponins, and phytosterols have been identified from chickweed, but there is virtually no scientific research on pharmacological and clinical aspects. Its best use is as a semi-wild spring green for salads.

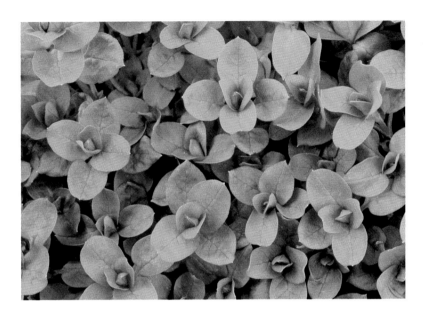

Used For:
Nutrition • Inflammation (topical)

Preparations:
Dried herb, whole or cut and sifted; capsules, tincture.

Typical Dosages:
Capsules: Up to nine 400–500 mg capsules a day.
Food: Eat fresh leaves and tender stems in the spring.
Tea: Steep 1 tsp dried herb in a cup of hot water for 10–15 minutes.
Tincture (1:5, 50% alcohol): 15–25 drops 3 times a day.
Or follow manufacturer's or practitioner's recommendations.

Cautions:
Chickweed itself is not associated with side effects; however, it may concentrate toxins in contaminated soil and has been known to be toxic to grazing cows.

Cranberry

Vaccinium macrocarpon

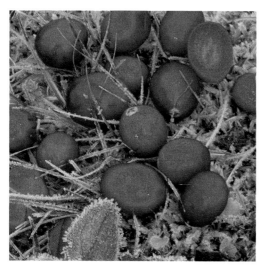

Source: A low-growing shrub of the heath family with leathery leaves and astringent red berries, cranberry is familiar to all, particularly in holiday sauces. It grows in bogs from Newfoundland to Manitoba south to Virginia and into the Midwest. Most commercial berries are produced in Massachusetts and Wisconsin.

Traditional Use: Cranberries and their juice are long-standing folk treatments for urinary infections. In early American medicine, the crushed berries were applied to tumors and poulticed on wounds. The berries were recognized as a treatment for scurvy (a vitamin C deficiency) and dysentery.

Current Use: Recent research shows that cranberry juice and cranberry extracts prevent adhesion of *E. coli* bacteria to the linings of the bladder and the gut, thereby inhibiting their ability to colonize and cause infection. A recent study of elderly patients found that 4 to 6 ounces of cranberry juice daily had a preventive, rather than a curative effect on urinary tract infections. In other studies the juice was effective as a urinary deodorant in bedridden patients with high levels of white blood cells and bacteria in the urine.

Most studies have involved cranberry juice. However, a recent

> Cranberries and their juice are long-standing folk treatments for urinary infections.

clinical study on powdered cranberry concentrate in capsules showed that they were effective in reducing the number of cases of urinary tract infections.

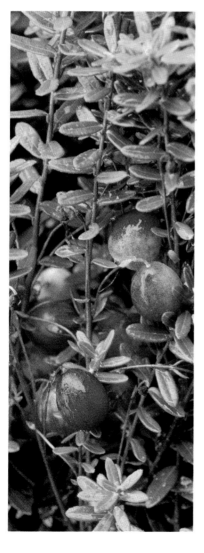

Used For:
Mild urinary tract infections

Preparations:
Whole fruit, raw or jellied; juice; fruit concentrate, capsules.

Typical Dosages:
Capsules: Up to nine 400–500 mg capsules a day. For intensive use, up to 15 capsules may be taken.
Food: 3–10 oz fresh fruit a day.
Juice: 5–20 oz cranberry juice cocktail a day.
Or follow manufacturer's or practitioner's recommendations.

Cautions:
If you suspect a urinary tract or kidney problem, see your doctor.

Damiana

Turnera diffusa

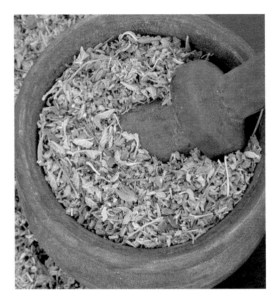

Sources: Damiana, a member of the *Turnera* family (Turneraceae), is a scraggly three-foot shrub native to warm regions of western Mexico. The dried aromatic leaves are used.

Traditional Use: Historically in western Mexico, damiana has been used as a beverage tea that can also treat colic, stop bed wetting, and bring on suppressed menses. Inhaling steam from the tea is said to relieve headache. Its longstanding reputation as an aphrodisiac evolves out of the first attempts to market the herb in the 1870s. Writing from La Paz, Mexico, in February, 1904, Professor John Uri Lloyd observed its use. "Damiana is a homely, domestic remedy, innocent of the attributes under which, in American medicine, it has, for a quarter of a century, been forced to masquerade." Nearly a century later, the controversy continues.

Current Use: Nearly all modern herb books mention the use of damiana as an aphrodisiac. As Lloyd pointed out, this resulted from the use of the term "damiana" on patent medicine preparations promoted as aphrodisiacs, whose other ingredients were not revealed. No reasonable scientific evidence confirms damiana's reputation as an aphrodisiac. An elixir and fluid extract of the herb were listed in the *National Formulary* from 1888 to 1916; the leaves and fluid extract were included up to 1947. Damiana was returned to use in the 1960s. No reasonable scientific evidence confirms its aphrodisiac qualities. Limited pharmacological studies do indicate possible antibacterial qualities, as well as the ability to lower blood sugar.

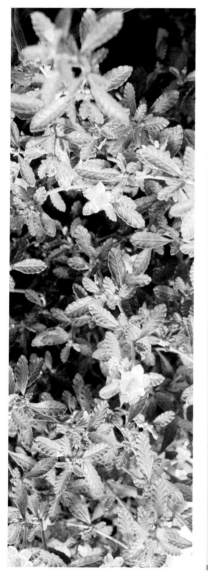

Used For:
Mild stimulant • Beverage tea • Aphrodisiac

Preparations:
Dried leaves; capsules, tinctures, other products.

Typical Dosages:
Capsules: Up to six 400-mg capsules a day.
Tea: Steep 1 tsp dried herb in a cup of hot water for 10–15 minutes up to 3 times a day.
Tincture (1:5, 60% alcohol): 20–60 drops in water 3 times a day.
Or follow manufacturer's or practitioner's recommendations.

Cautions:
No side effects or other adverse reactions to damiana are generally reported in the literature. Given damiana's long history of use in Mexico, predating the Spanish invasion, safety seems established. However, lacking toxicological studies, it, like all herbs, should be used in moderation.

Dandelion

Taraxacum officinale

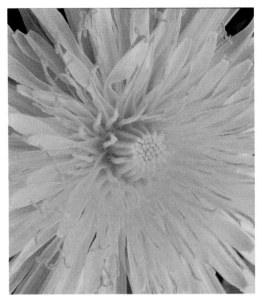

Source: Besides culinary use as coffee substitute and salad ingredient, the root and leaf of this pervasive weed of the aster family are also used in traditional medicine. Dandelion is grown commercially in both the United States and Europe.

Traditional Use: Both dandelion leaf and root have been used for centuries to treat liver, gallbladder, and kidney ailments, weak digestion, and rheumatism. They are also considered mildly laxative. The fresh root or its preparations are thought to be more potent than the dried root. The leaves have traditionally been used as a diuretic.

Current Use: Dandelion root and leaf are widely used in herbal medicines in Europe. The leaves are diuretic but also high in potassium, so they help to compensate for the potassium lost with increased urination. Bitter compounds in the leaves (and root) have increased bile secretion in laboratory animals by more than 40 percent. The leaves are prescribed as a diuretic in cases of water retention and for bloating accompanied by flatulence and loss of appetite.

The bitter compounds in dandelion root help stimulate digestion and are mildly laxative. The roots have been shown to be moderately anti-inflammatory, supporting their traditional use in the treatment of rheumatism. The root is used for dyspepsia, loss of appetite, as a diuretic, and for disorders associated with inhibited bile secretion from the liver.

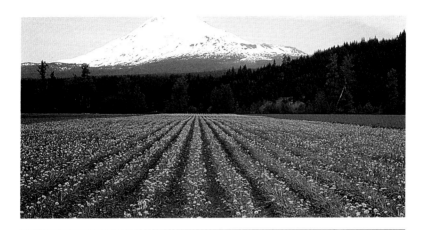

Used For:
Stimulating appetite • Diuresis • Increasing bile flow

Preparations:
Fresh or dried leaves and root; capsules, liquid extracts, tablets, tinctures. Extracts in 25% alcohol are best for increasing bile flow.

Typical Dosages:
Food: Eat young leaves raw or lightly cooked in the spring.
Dried herb: 3–9 tsp 3 times a day.
Liquid extract (1:1, 45% alcohol): 30–60 drops 3 times a day.
Tea: Steep 1–2 tsp cut-and-sifted dried root in a cup of hot water for 10–15 minutes. Take twice a day, in morning and evening. Or follow manufacturer's or practitioner's recommendations.

Cautions:
The German Commission E monographs on dandelion leaf and root indicate that in cases of gallstones, dandelion products should be used only under a physician's supervision. If bile ducts are obstructed, dandelion should not be used at all. The milky latex in fresh dandelion leaves may cause contact dermatitis. The bitterness of dandelion root may cause hyperacidity in some individuals.

Devil's Claw

Harpagophytum procumbens

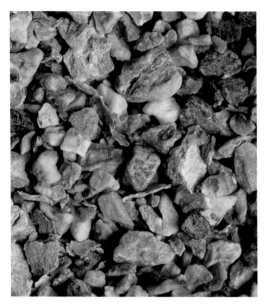

Sources: Devil's claw, also known as grapple plant, is a shrubby vine in the pedalium family native to southwest Africa. The fruits have large woody grapples (hence the name grapple plant) that disperse seed by sticking in animal fur. Occasionally, these barbed fruits can become stuck in a foot or hoof, or hook themselves into the mouth of a grazing animal. The secondary tubers are the principal plant part used. Most commercial supplies are wild-harvested from the Kalahari deserts and savannas of Namibia.

Traditional Use: The tubers were highly prized by African Bushmen, Hottentots, and Bantu as a bitter tonic for indigestion. A tea was also used for fever, as a blood purifier, and to relieve rheumatic and arthritic pain. In various African cultures a small amount of the tuber was given near delivery of a baby to help relieve the mother's pain. An ointment of the fresh tuber was applied to the abdomen of women anticipating a difficult birth. Externally, it was also used for boils, sores, ulcers, and as a folk cancer remedy.

Current Use: Preparations of the tuber were introduced into European phytomedicine in the early 1950s, based on the herb's reputation as an anti-inflammatory for rheumatism and arthritis. The secondary tubers contain twice as much of the perceived active component, harpagoside, as the primary root. While devil's claw products are standardized to this compound, studies have shown that other components are involved in its pain-relieving qualities. Animal and human studies have confirmed anti-inflammatory activity, though clinical trials have given mixed results on the herb's effectiveness for relieving inflammatory pain. A recent controlled clinical trial involving 118 patients showed positive, though inconclusive, results in reducing or eliminating acute attacks of low back pain. Various animal studies have shown that extracts of the tubers may act on heart muscles. In Germany, preparations are approved for treating loss of appetite, indigestion, and inflammatory joint conditions.

Used For:
Inflammation • Pain relief • Indigestion

Preparations:
Dried secondary tubers, cut and sifted or powdered; capsules, tablets, tinctures, tea. Some products are standardized to harpagoside content.

Typical Dosages:
Capsules: Up to six 400–500 mg capsules a day.
Tea: For indigestion, steep 1/4 tsp of dried tuber in a cup of hot water for 10–15 minutes.
Tincture: 30 drops 3 times a day.
Or follow manufacturer's or practitioner's recommendations.

Cautions:
According to the German health authorities, use is contraindicated when gastric or duodenal ulcers are present. Animal studies have shown the tuber to have relatively low toxicity. Given its potential effect on the heart muscle, it should be used cautiously and under medical supervision if heart disease is present. Avoid use during pregnancy and lactation.

Dong-quai
Angelica sinensis

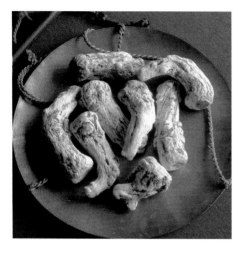

Source: Dong-quai is the dried root of a member of the parsley family. The plant thrives in high, cool, shaded mountain woods in southern and western China. Most of the supply is commercially grown there, rather than wild-harvested.

Traditional Use: The name dong-quai means "proper order." Used in China for thousands of years, it is regarded as highly as ginseng. In Traditional Chinese Medicine, the root is believed to return the system to proper order by nourishing the blood and helping harmonize vital energy. In China it is one of the more frequently prescribed herbs and appears in prescriptions (with other herbs) for abnormal or suppressed menstruation, anemia, and other conditions. In the West, it is used to tone and regulate the female reproductive system and is prescribed for premenstrual syndrome (PMS), menstrual difficulties, and menopause symptoms.

Current Use: Most research on the plant has been done in China and Japan since the early 1960s. Experiments show that whereas the root's volatile oil causes relaxation of the uterine muscle, both water and alcohol extracts stimulate uterine contractions; alcohol extracts are stronger. Dong-quai also normalizes irregular uterine contractions and improves blood flow to the uterus. The actions do not appear to result from estrogenic activity, because dong-quai does not produce changes in the ovaries or vaginal tissue. It has been shown to improve circulation and lower blood pressure by increasing blood flow in the peripheral vessels and reducing vascular resistance. Experiments have also confirmed that it reduces inflammation, pain, and spasms, and increases the number of red blood cells and platelets. A recent study found that dong-quai could help improve protein metabolism in patients with kidney disease. Animal studies have also confirmed that dong-quai protects the liver from toxins and helps it to utilize more oxygen. Most clinical studies in China and Japan have involved dong-quai in combination with other herbs, so their generally positive results in treating gynecological problems are difficult to assess for dong-quai alone.

Used For:
Menstrual difficulties • Menopausal difficulties • PMS

Preparations:
Dried root, whole, sliced, or powdered; capsules, tablets, tinctures, combination products.

Typical Dosages:
Capsules: Up to six 500–600 mg capsules a day.
Tincture (1:5, 70% alcohol): 5–20 drops up to 3 times a day.
Or follow manufacturer's or practitioner's recommendations.

Cautions:
Pregnant or nursing women should avoid dong quai unless supervised by a qualified medical practitioner. In TCM, it is not given to patients with diarrhea, because it is considered somewhat laxative.

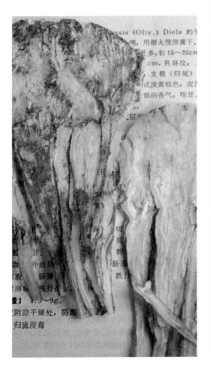

Echinacea

Echinacea angustifolia, E. pallida, E. purpurea

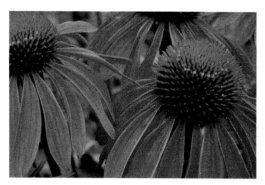

Sources: Echinacea, also known as purple coneflower, is the root or aboveground parts (harvested in flower) of three species of large, robust daisylike plants of the aster family. *E. angustifolia* and *E. pallida* are harvested from the prairies of the midwestern United States. Some commercial cultivation of these two species has developed as they have become more scarce in the wild. *E. purpurea,* also native to the Midwest, is the most widely used species of the three. The entire world supply is cultivated.

Traditional Use: Native Americans of the prairie used echinacea for more medicinal purposes than they did any other plant, for everything from colds to cancer. It entered formal medicine in 1895, becoming the best-selling American medicinal plant prescribed by physicians into the 1920s. Later replaced by antibiotics in the United States, it has enjoyed continuous popularity in Europe. In 1993 German physicians prescribed echinacea more than 2.5 million times. Traditionally, herbalists consider it a blood purifier and aid to fighting infections.

Current Use: Today most consumers use echinacea to prevent and treat colds and to help heal infections. Echinacea enhances the particle-ingestion capacity of white blood cells and other specialized immune-system cells, increasing their ability to attack foreign invaders such as cold or flu viruses. Besides stimulating a healthy immune system to deal more effectively with invading viruses, echinacea helps accelerate healing if infection already exists.

A 1992 German double-blind, placebo-controlled study of 180 volunteers using *E. purpurea* found that a dose of 4 droppers of tincture (equivalent to 900 mg of dried root) decreased symptoms and duration of flu-like infections. The best-studied form of echinacea is a preparation made from the fresh expressed juice of *E. purpurea*. No single chemical component has been identified as causing echinacea's medicinal action. A 1997 controlled clinical study on 120 volunteers in Sweden showed that daily treatment with the juice of fresh flowering *E. purpurea* at the first sign of cold symptoms inhibited development of colds, and if a cold was in progress, it cut the duration in half. More clinical studies are needed to determine clear therapeutic indications, the best preparations, and the most effective dosage.

Used For:
Colds • Flu • Minor infections

Preparations:
Dried whole herb or root; capsules, expressed juice of fresh flowering plant, flex-tabs, tablets, tinctures. Some products are standardized to echinacoside despite the fact the compound has not been found to stimulate the immune system.

Typical Dosages:
Capsules: Up to nine 300–400 mg capsules a day.
Tincture: 60 drops 3 times a day. This is equivalent to 1 g of dried root a day. Use as needed at the onset of symptoms of cold or flu. Take continuously for two weeks, followed by a resting period of one week.
Or follow manufacturer's or practitioner's recommendations.

Cautions:
Persons who are allergic to the pollen of other members of the aster family, such as ragweed, may also be allergic to echinacea. The German government recommends that nonspecific immunostimulants, including echinacea, should not be used in cases of impaired immune response involving diseases of the immune system itself, including tuberculosis, multiple sclerosis, and HIV infection. This finding is based on the concept that immunostimulants should not be used when autoimmune disease is present.

Elderberry

Sambucus canadensis (North American elderberry)
S. nigra (European or black elderberry)

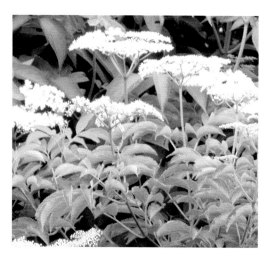

Sources: Elderberry comes from several of the nine species of the genus *Sambucus* in the honeysuckle family, particularly elder flower and fruit from the North American *S. canadensis* and the European *S. nigra*. The American elder ranges from British Columbia to Nova Scotia, south to the mountains of North Carolina, and west to Arizona. The European elderberry occurs throughout Europe, except for extreme northern areas, and is widely cultivated for its edible fruits.

Traditional Use: American herbal traditions combined the dried flowers of *S. canadensis* with peppermint for treating fevers and colds. The flowers, fruits, bark, and leaves have all been used as folk remedies by Native Americans. Tea from the inner bark was used as a diuretic and strong laxative, as well as to induce vomiting. Black elderberry has long been used in European folk medicine, like its American counterpart, for treating colds and fevers. The fruits have been used as a mild laxative and diuretic, and to induce sweating.

Current Use: Most chemical research on elderberry has involved black elderberry, and current interest in black elderberry extract stems from the research of an Israeli scientist, Dr. Madeleine Mumcuoglu. Dr. Mumcuoglu and colleagues at Hadassah University Medical Center in Jerusalem developed an elderberry extract standardized to contain three flavonoids. The preparation was used in a clinical study during a flu outbreak in Israel in 1993; the extract reduced the severity and duration of flu symptoms compared to a placebo in a limited population sampling. Sold under the trade name Sambucol™, the extract's effective compounds inhibit the ability of the flu virus to enter cells, thereby disarming the virus's infection capability.

The flowers of elderberry are the subject of a positive German therapeutic monograph and are allowed to be used to induce sweating in cases of fevers (diaphoretic), as well as to increase bronchial secretion in the treatment of colds.

Used For:
Fruits: Prevention and treatment of colds and flu
Flowers: Colds, fevers, bronchitis

Preparations:
Dried flowers or berries of European or American elder, whole or powdered; capsules, tablets, tinctures, and other products.

Typical Dosages:
Capsules: Up to six 500–600 mg capsules a day.
Syrup: Simmer 3 tsp dried fruit in 1 pint water. Sweeten with honey to taste. In the case of commercial preparations, follow manufacturer's instructions.
Tea: Simmer 2–3 tsp dried flowers in hot water for 10–15 minutes. Use up to 3 times a day.
Tincture: 40 drops every 4 hours.
Or follow manufacturer's or practitioner's recommendations.

Cautions:
Safe use of elder always relates to the dried or cooked flowers and fruits. When fresh, all plant parts can produce allergic or other adverse reactions. There are reports in the literature of children developing symptoms from handling toys made from fresh elder stems. Since the stems have a large soft pith (up to 90 percent the diameter of the stem) children have used them for making pea shooters or whistles, and some children have shown reactions.

Eleuthero

Eleutherococcus senticosus

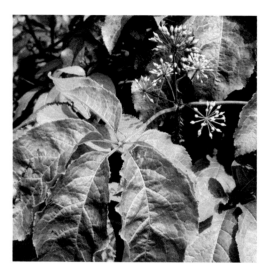

Source: Eleuthero, also known as Siberian ginseng, is the root, root bark, or stem of a shrub in the ginseng family. It grows in thickets in northeast China, eastern Russia, Korea, and Japan's northern island, Hokkaido. Most of the supply comes from Siberia and China, but it is also grown in eastern Europe. The Chinese call it *ci-wu-jia*.

Traditional Use: For more than 2,000 years, Eleuthero has been used in China for invigorating vital energy (Qi), normalizing body functions, improving health, promoting good appetite, and helping to assure a long life. Generally, it serves as a preventive medicine and general tonic.

> **Generally, eleuthero serves as a preventive medicine and general tonic.**

Current Use: I. I. Brekhman, the leading Russian researcher on ginseng, has described eleuthero as an "adaptogen," an innocuous substance that causes minimal disorders of an organism's function. It must have a "nonspecific action" that normalizes body functions, no matter what the condition or disease. Adaptogens are essentially general tonics.

Studies done since the early 1950s have shown that eleuthero extract increases mental alertness, work output, and the quality of work under stressful conditions and in athletic performance. In addition, it strongly stimulates the immune system.

German authorities allow eleuthero to be labeled as an invigorating tonic for fatigue, convalescence, decreased work capacity, or difficulty in concentration.

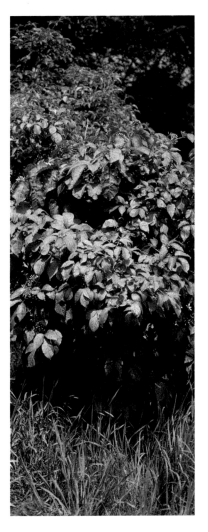

Used For:
Improving well-being and acuity • Immunostimulant

Preparations:
Dried roots or stems, powdered; capsules, tablets, tinctures.

Typical Dosages:
Capsules: Up to nine 400–500 mg capsules a day.
Tincture (1:5, 60% alcohol): 20 drops up to 3 times a day. Or follow manufacturer's or practitioner's recommendations.

Cautions:
No side effects are reported for eleuthero. While the German Commission E notes that people with high blood pressure should avoid eleuthero, there does not appear to be good clinical evidence to support this caution.

Ephedra

Ephedra sinica, E. intermedia, E. equisetina

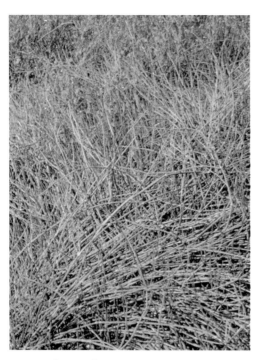

Sources: The Chinese herb *ma-huang*, known in the West as ephedra, is the dried stem of three species of primitive shrubs in the ephedra family found in desert regions around the world. Three species are commonly used as source plants: *E. sinica, E. intermedia,* and *E. equisetina,* all native to the steppes of north and northwestern China. The nine species and two hybrids that are native to North American deserts do not contain the alkaloids the Asian species do.

Traditional Use: Ephedra is first mentioned in *Shen Nong Ben Cao Jing,* a list of 365 herbs from the first century A.D. In Traditional Chinese Medicine, its functions are to induce sweat, soothe breath, and promote urination. Ephedra has been used for more than 2,000 years to treat bronchial asthma, colds and flu, chills, lack of perspiration, headache, nasal congestion, aching joints and bones, cough and wheezing, and edema.

Current Use: Ephedra's alkaloids ephedrine and pseudoephedrine stimulate the central nervous system and heart muscle, dilate the bronchial tubes, and elevate blood pressure. Both natural ephedrine and pseudoephedrine from ma-huang and synthetic forms of the alkaloids are sold commercially in over-the-counter bronchodilators for mild seasonal or chronic asthma. The alkaloids are also found in products to relieve sinusitis and nasal congestion. Pseudoephedrine's effects are somewhat weaker than those of ephedrine. Ephedra also has diuretic and anti-inflammatory activity.

A discussion of the side effects of this herb or its alkaloids when abused could fill a small book. Some of the known effects include insomnia, motor disturbances, high blood pressure, glaucoma, impaired cerebral circulation, and urinary disturbances. Ephedrine-containing products should not be used by anyone who has hypertension, high blood pressure, heart disease, thyroid disease, or diabetes, or who is taking a monoamine oxidase inhibitor. Abuse of ephedra-alkaloid products combined with caffeine has lead to at least 22 deaths and over 800 reports of adverse reactions, prompting the Food and Drug Administration to contemplate regulatory action such as restricting use of the alkaloids to legitimate over-the-counter drug preparations.

Used For:
Mild asthma • Nasal congestion

Preparations:
Dried stems; capsules, tablets, teas, tinctures.

Typical Dosage:
Tincture: 15–30 drops in water up to 4 times a day.
Or follow manufacturer's or practitioner's recommendations; observe Cautions below.

Cautions:
See "Current Use" for the extensive cautions associated with this herb. Over-the-counter drugs containing ephedra alkaloids are required to carry a warning against exceeding the recommended dose (except under a physician's direction). Also, if symptoms worsen or are not relieved in an hour, discontinue use immediately and seek a physician's advice. It is best to seek the opinion of a physician before using ephedra products.

Evening Primrose

Oenothera biennis

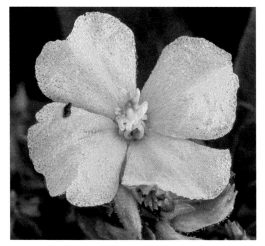

Source: Evening primrose oil is obtained from the seeds of a common wildflower of the evening primrose family native to eastern North America and widely naturalized in Europe and western North America. Most seed for oil production is grown commercially.

Traditional Use: Native Americans gathered the seeds for food in Utah and Nevada. Those in eastern North America used the whole plant as a poultice for bruises and a tea to treat obesity; they used a decoction of the root to treat hemorrhoids. Early settlers used the leaves to treat wounds and to soothe sore throats and upset stomach. Use of the seed oil is relatively recent.

> ## Use of the seed oil of evening primrose is relatively recent.

Current Use: Used as a dietary supplement, evening primrose oil provides essential fatty acids, especially gamma-linolenic acid (GLA). Factors such as aging, alcohol abuse, cancerous conditions, poor dietary habits, or improper nutrition may cause essential-fatty-acid deficiencies, which can be mitigated with dietary supplementation of GLA from evening primrose oil. More than 120 studies in fifteen countries report potential use of the oil in treating asthma, migraine, inflammation, premenstrual syndrome (PMS), diabetes, arthritis, and alcoholism. Conflicting results point to the need for further well-designed scientific studies.

On the other hand, over a dozen clinical studies have registered positive results for the use of evening primrose oil in the treatment of allergy-induced eczema. German authorities allow a daily dose of 500 mg of evening primrose oil in the treatment of atopic eczema, reducing symptoms such as inflammation and dryness, and improving overall skin health. It is also approved for eczema in England.

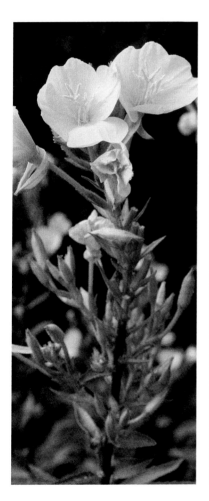

Used For:
Allergy-induced eczema • Essential fatty acids deficiencies • PMS symptoms

Preparations:
Expressed oil from seeds; capsules.

Typical Dosages:
Capsules: Up to 12 capsules of oil a day.
Oil: 1/2 tsp a day.
Or follow manufacturer's or practitioner's recommendations.

Cautions:
No known contraindications or drug interactions have been reported for evening primrose oil. In clinical studies, fewer than 2 percent of patients taking it for long periods reported side effects such as abdominal discomfort, nausea, and headache.

Eyebright

Euphrasia officinalis

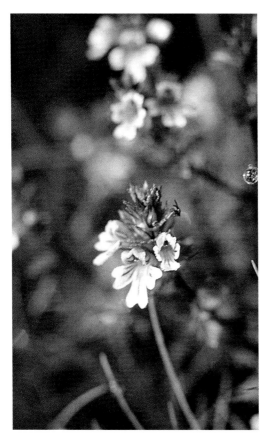

Sources: The genus *Euphrasia* in the figwort family is a complex plant group with at least 170 named species, many separated by minute technical details (microspecies). *E. officinalis* is the representative name most often used in the literature. Occurring in cold temperate regions, the herb of this small plant, scarcely 6" tall, is used. *Euphrasia* species are hemiparasitic, that is, their roots attach to those of grasses to derive some of their nutrients.

Traditional Use: The name alone bespeaks the primary use of the herb through history—a wash or tea taken internally for treatment of eye diseases. The bright, small, showy flower, suggesting an eye, is the source of its common name and use, based on the medieval doctrine of signatures. The flowers have tiny stripes, like bloodshot eyes, which sparked its use in European folk traditions for conjunctivitis and blepharitis. It has also been used as a cold compress for treatment of eye fatigue and sties.

Current Use: Despite centuries of use for the treatment of eye ailments, current research on eyebright can be summed up in a phrase: "precious little." Its chemistry has been relatively well-studied, however, and includes flavonoids, iridoids, tannins, and a small amount of a volatile oil; some of these compounds have antibacterial and anti-inflammatory effects. A recent study looked at the herb's ability to kill cells, exploring its potential as a source of anti-cancer agents. The results were negative. No animal or human studies have been published. There is no scientific evidence to support use of the herb, but then, no scientific research has been conducted.

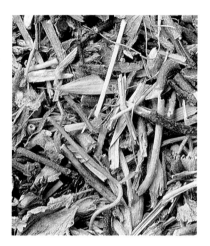

Used For:
Folk medicine for eye ailments

Preparations:
Dried herb, whole, cut and sifted, or powdered; capsules, tablets, tinctures, other preparations.

Typical Dosages:
Capsules: Up to five 400–500 mg capsules a day.
Tea: Steep 2–3 tsp in a cup of hot water for 10–15 minutes. Use 3 times a day. May be used externally as an eye wash or compress.
Tincture: 30–40 drops up to 4 times a day.
Or follow manufacturer's or practitioner's recommendations.

Cautions:
Given the fact that there are virtually no human or animal studies on the use of the herb and its safety, the application of preparations to the eyes should be approached very cautiously. Such preparations must be free from bacteria, in order not to introduce infection into the eyes. Preparations are best applied by a qualified herbal practitioner.

Fennel

Foeniculum vulgare

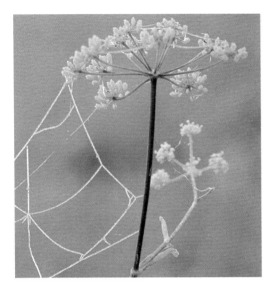

Sources: Fennel is a member of the parsley family, native to the Mediterranean region. It is widely naturalized in other parts of the world, and especially common in California. Different varieties of fennel are grown for their thickened edible celery-like stems, with a sweet anise flavor, the anise-flavored leaves, and the fruits ("seeds") used both for flavoring and medicinal purposes. Major producers include China, Egypt, and several eastern European countries. Several varieties are cultivated. *F. vulgare* var. *dulce,* sweet fennel, is grown for the fruits and their essential oil. *F. vulgare* var. *azoricum,* is finnochio or Florence fennel, grown as a vegetable for its swollen stems. *F. vulgare* var. *vulgare,* bitter fennel, is also grown for its fruits.

> **Fennel is mentioned in virtually every European work on herbal medicines from ancient times to the present day.**

Traditional Use: Fennel is mentioned in virtually every European work on herbal medicines from ancient times to the present day. The ancient Romans grew the herb for its edible shoots and the aromatic seeds. In the ninth century, Charlemagne encouraged its cultivation in central Europe. Though native to southern Europe, it was used in Anglo-Saxon folk medicine by the eleventh century. For hundreds of years, the seeds have been valued as a digestive carminative, stimulant, and mild diuretic; they have been used to treat fevers and stimulate milk flow. A primary use is to mask the bad flavor of medicines. The seeds were official in the *United States Pharmacopoeia* from 1820 to 1970.

Current Use: Fennel seed is approved in Germany for treating digestive problems such as bloating, flatulence, and mild spasms of the gastrointestinal tract. Fennel syrup is used for catarrhs of the upper respiratory tract. Studies have confirmed antimicrobial, antispasmodic, and anti-inflammatory activity. Boiled-water extracts of the leaves have been shown to produce a significant reduction in arterial blood pressure without affecting the heart rate or respiratory rate, while nonboiled water extracts had no effect. Research starting in the 1930s looked at fennel seed oil as a potential source of synthetic estrogens, given the herb's reputation to increase milk secretion, promote menstruation, and increase libido. This research is ongoing.

Used For:
Stomach bloating • Digestive spasms • Catarrh

Preparations:
Whole seed, capsules, tinctures.

Typical Dosages:
Capsules: Up to three 400–500 mg capsules a day, or follow manufacturer's or practitioner's recommendations.
Tea: Simmer 2–3 tsp crushed seed in a cup of hot water for 10–15 minutes. Use 1 time a day.
Tincture (1:5, 60% alcohol): 30–60 drops in water up to 4 times a day.
Or follow manufacturer's or practitioner's recommendations.

Cautions:
Rare allergic skin or respiratory-tract reactions have been reported. Given a potential estrogenic effect, avoid during pregnancy.

Fenugreek

Trigonella foenum-graecum

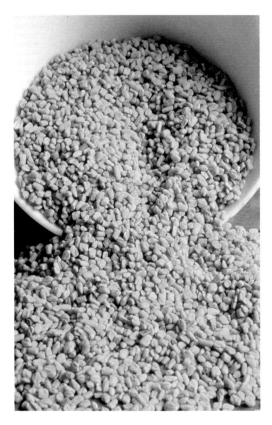

Sources: Fenugreek, a member of the pea family, is an ancient herb native to southern Europe and southwest Asia, and cultivated in warm climates throughout the world. The plant has been grown since the time of the Assyrians, and the seed was found in the tomb of Tutankhamun. India and China are primary producers of fenugreek.

Traditional Use: Described as carminative, tonic, and aphrodisiac, the mucilaginous seeds have been used as both food and medicine for millennia. As food the seeds are eaten raw or cooked, used in curries in India, in bread in Egypt, and as a coffee substitute in Africa. They have also been used to stimulate milk flow. In his *CRC Handbook of Medicinal Herbs* (1985), Dr. James A. Duke mentions that harem women in Arab countries consumed the seeds to promote buxomness. The leaves are considered to have cooling qualities and a tea is used to soothe inflammation of the intestinal tract.

Current Use: Fenugreek seeds are approved by the German health authorities internally for treating loss of appetite (anorexia) and externally as a poultice for local inflammation. In other European herbal traditions, fenugreek is used as a mild laxative, for dyspepsia and gastritis, as a nutritive tea for convalescents, and as an expectorant.

Traditional use for diabetes has prompted numerous animal and a few human studies. In a recent clinical trial on the use of the herb to lower cholesterol in patients with non-insulin dependent diabetes, significant reductions in low-density lipoproteins were observed, an effect attributed to the seeds' gel fiber. Other studies have found that fenugreek seed lowers blood sugar.

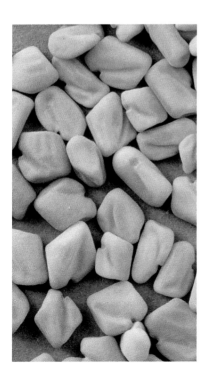

Used For:
Gastritis • Excess cholesterol • Nutrition

Preparations:
Seed, whole or powdered; capsules, tablets.

Typical Dosages:
Capsules: Up to six 600–700 mg capsules a day.
Seed: 1½ tsp a day. For external use, soak 10 tsp powdered seed in hot water to make a poultice. Or follow manufacturer's or practitioner's recommendations.

Cautions:
No side effects or contraindications are generally reported, though in clinical studies, some patients have experienced intestinal gas and diarrhea. Diabetic patients should be warned that use of fenugreek may interfere with other therapies. With a high content of mucilagin, the seeds may coat the stomach and prevent absorption of other drugs. Given uterine-stimulant activity and a possible estrogenic effect, use during pregnancy should be avoided.

Feverfew

Tanacetum parthenium (formerly *Chrysanthemum parthenium*)

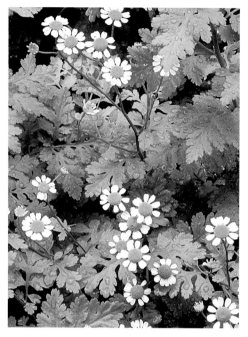

Source: Feverfew is the fresh or dried leaf of a member of the aster family native to the Balkan peninsula. It is naturalized in Europe and North and South America.

Traditional Use: The English herbalist Nicholas Culpeper (1787) wrote that feverfew "is very effectual for all pains in the head coming of a cold cause, the herb being bruised and applied to the crown of the head." For more than 2,000 years, feverfew has been a folk medicine taken internally for fevers, headache, or menstrual regulation, or applied externally to relieve pain.

Current Use: Modern use of feverfew focuses on migraine prevention. A compound called parthenolide (not found in all feverfew varieties) appears to be responsible for the anti-migraine effects.

When a research group in England asked for volunteers with experience using feverfew, it received an astonishing 25,500 replies. Of the 300 subjects interviewed, 70 percent of those eating one to three fresh leaves a day reported a reduction in migraine frequency or pain. In a 1985 double-blind study conducted by London researchers, seventeen patients ingested an average daily dose of 60 mg of feverfew leaves and experienced no change in frequency or severity of migraine symptoms. Those who took a placebo, however, had an increase in the frequency and severity of headaches, nausea, and vomiting.

In a 1988 randomized, double-blind, placebo-controlled, crossover study in Nottingham, seventy-two volunteers received either a feverfew capsule or a placebo daily for four months. The feverfew treatment was associated with a reduction in the frequency and severity of migraines and related vomiting, but the duration was not significantly shortened.

A study by a Dutch research group published in 1996 found that a feverfew extract produced in the laboratory had no significant benefits compared with placebo. On the other hand, an Israeli research group has recently published a new clinical study on the preventive use of feverfew against migraine in fifty-seven patients over four months. The authors concluded this study provides convincing proof that the feverfew preparations can profoundly reduce the pain, nausea, and sensitivity to noise and light typically associated with migraine attacks.

Used For:
Migraine headaches

Preparations:
Fresh or dried leaves; capsules, tablets, tinctures. Some products are standardized to 0.2% parthenolide, though other constituents may be responsible for the herb's action.

Typical Dosages:
Capsules: Up to three 300–400 mg capsules a day, or follow manufacturer's or practitioner's recommendations.
Fresh herb: Eat 2 average-sized leaves a day.
Tincture: 15–30 drops a day.
Or follow manufacturer's or practitioner's recommendations.

Cautions: No long-term studies have been done on feverfew's safety. As many as 7 to 12 percent of patients using feverfew have reported mouth ulcers, tongue inflammation, swelling of the lips, and occasional loss of taste. These symptoms disappear when use is stopped. Avoid during pregnancy.

Flaxseed

Linum usitatissimum

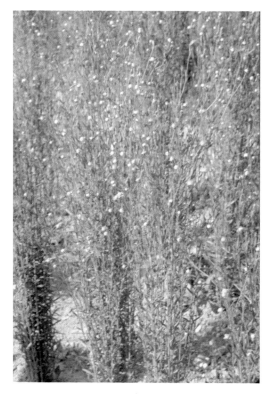

Sources: A member of the flax family, flaxseed is one of the world's older cultivated plants, grown for its fiber (linen), seed oil (linseed oil), and seeds, which have been used in pharmacy for centuries. The plant occurs throughout much of the world; commercial supplies come from North Africa, Turkey, Argentina, and Canada.

Traditional Use: Use in Egypt dates as far back as the twenty-third century B.C. Greeks of the seventh century B.C. ate roasted seeds. The oily, mucilaginous properties of the seed are mentioned by early Roman authors, who reported flaxseed's use for colds, urinary tract inflammations, and lung conditions.

Current Use: In modern phytomedicine, the seeds are used as a mild, lubricating laxative, and to relieve irritable bowel syndrome, diverticulitis, gastritis, and enteritis. Flaxseed is also used to correct problems caused from abuse of stimulant laxatives. Unaffected by stomach acid, the mucilaginous fiber in the seeds absorbs water in the colon, increasing volume and softening stools. The mucilage in flaxseed is not damaged by stomach acid or by the alkaline conditions of the small intestine. It has been shown to increase intestinal peristalsis and relieve pain from inflammatory intestinal conditions. There is a latent period of several days before effects are observed. A flaxseed poultice is used to allay pain of skin inflammations.

Flaxseed oil is high in omega-3 fatty acids and is widely promoted in the American market as a dietary supplement. The seeds contain lignans that bind to estrogenic receptors and may have positive benefits in women with ovarian dysfunction. The seeds may also reduce the risk of breast and colon cancer.

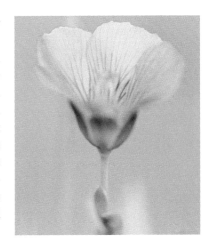

Used For:
Constipation • Irritable bowel syndrome • Source of omega-3 essential fatty acids • Chemoprevention

Preparation:
Seed, whole or powdered; expressed oil of seed.

Typical Dosage:
Seed: Soak 1/2–1 tbsp whole or cracked seed in 1 cup water. Use up to 3 times a day.
Or follow manufacturer's or practitioner's recommendations.

Cautions: Use is contraindicated in colicky bowel conditions or if obstructions of the bowels are suspected. While flaxseed does contain cyanide compounds, several studies have shown that even large single doses (up to 100 g) produce no significant increase in blood levels of cyanide. Use is generally considered to be safe.

Fo-ti

Polygonum multiflorum

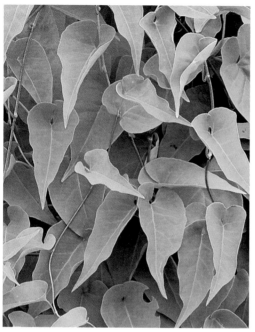

Source: Fo-ti is the dried or cured root of a twining vine in the knotweed family, found in most regions of China. It is also occasionally grown in American gardens as an ornamental. The plant's name was bestowed in the early 1970s by an American herb marketer; in China, it is known as *he-shou-wu*.

Traditional Use: In Chinese medicine the dried (unprocessed) root and the cured (processed) root are considered two different herbs. The unprocessed root is used to relax the bowels and detoxify the blood. The processed root is used to strengthen the blood, invigorate the liver and kidneys, and supplement vital energy (Qi). Processed fo-ti is one of the more widely-used tonics in Traditional Chinese Medicine (TCM), which employs it to enhance longevity, increase vigor, and promote fertility. It is also an ingredient in TCM formulas for premature gray hair, low back pain, angina pectoris, low energy, and other conditions.

Current Use: In animals, the processed root reduces blood cholesterol. The root contains lectins, which appear to help prevent cholesterol accumulation in the liver and fat retention in the blood. Animal experiments show that fo-ti can help reduce formation of plaque and fat deposits on arterial walls. It also inhibits the growth of bacteria, increases laboratory animals' ability to adapt to cold temperatures, and promotes the formation of red blood cells. An extract of the processed root has shown antitumor, antioxidant, and immunostimulant effects in animals.

Unprocessed roots lubricate the bowels, producing a laxative effect. Several clinical studies in China suggest the processed herb is useful in treating high cholesterol, heart conditions, and chronic bronchitis. Mounting evidence supports fo-ti's traditional use as a tonic.

Used For:
Tonic • Building blood • Lowering cholesterol

Preparations:
Dried root, whole, sliced, or powdered; capsules, tablets, tinctures. Processed root, as used in Chinese medicine, is dark reddish brown; unprocessed root is light brown to brown. Processing changes the action of the herb.

Typical Dosages:
Capsules: Up to six 600–700 mg capsules a day, or follow manufacturer's or practitioner's recommendations.
Tea: Soak 1–3 tsp dried root in 1 cup hot water for 10–15 minutes.
Tincture: 15–30 drops 3 times a day.
Or follow manufacturer's or practitioner's recommendations.

Cautions:
The unprocessed root can cause loose stools or diarrhea, sometimes with intestinal pain and nausea. The unprocessed root is considered potentially more toxic than the processed form. One case of allergic reaction to the cured root has been reported, although this form of fo-ti is considered minimally toxic when taken in proper doses. Large doses have resulted in numbness of the extremities and skin rashes.

Garcinia

Garcinia cambogia, G. indica

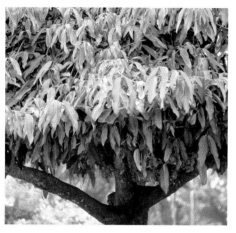

Sources: *Garcinia* is a genus of over 200 species of evergreen trees or shrubs in the garcinia family found in tropical Asia, Africa, and Polynesia. About thirty species are found in India alone, including *G. cambogia* and *G. indica,* which grow also in China and southeast Asia. *G. cambogia* has been called "Malabar tamarind," a misnomer, as the fruit should not be confused with tamarind (*Tamarindus indica*). The fruits of the two trees have a similar acidic flavor, typical of citric acid.

Traditional Use: The fruits have long been used as a food in India, especially on the west coast. Muslim populations in Laos, Malaysia, Thailand, and Burma use the fruits as a flavoring in curries and as a substitute for limes or tamarind. An extract of dried garcinia is traditionally taken after lamb dishes with a high fat content to aid in digestion. In folk traditions in India, the dried fruit rind has been decocted for rheumatism and bowel complaints.

> Various studies have shown that the principal acid in garcinia fruits produced significant reduction in food intake and body weight gain in rats.

Current Use: Starting in the late 1960s, various studies showed that, (—)-hydoxycitrate ((—)-HCA), the principal acid in garcinia fruits, produced significant reduction in food intake and body weight gain in rats. (—)-

HCA is considered a powerful inhibitor of fat accumulation, modifying the conversion of carbohydrates to fat in mammals. Other rat studies have shown garcinia to have an appetite-suppressant effect. However, the effect of (—)-HCA is different in lean rats and obese rats. One study found that in obese rats, while (—)-HCA produced a reduction in food intake and body weight, it did not reduce the percentage of body fat or the size of fat cells. Questions raised by these results will have to be answered by further studies.

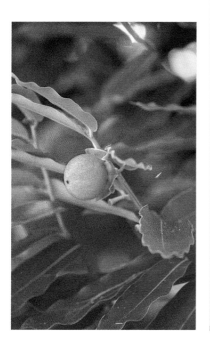

Used For:
Weight loss

Preparations:
Extracts of fruit, manufactured in India.

Typical Dosage:
Commercial products typically deliver 250 mg of (—)-HCA, a garcinia derivative, a day. It is often combined with chromium picolinate. Follow manufacturer's recommendations.

Cautions:
Garcinia has been used continuously and safely for centuries as a food. Problems associated with acute or chronic toxicity from eating the fruit are lacking. Garcinia alters lipid and carbohydrate metabolism. Unlike plant-based stimulants like ephedra or products containing caffeine, both of which have been used in the past in weight loss formulations, garcinia does not stimulate the central nervous system to burn calories. Clinically obese patients should discuss use of garcinia products with their health-care professional.

Garlic

Allium sativum

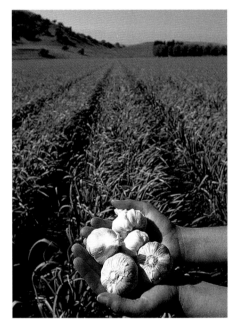

Source: No herb is so closely tied to the human experience as garlic. A member of the lily family, the bulb is unknown in the wild, having evolved under cultivation during the past 5,000 years.

Traditional Use: Garlic has been used as food and medicine since the age of the Egyptian pharaohs. The Greek historian and traveler Herodotus (484–425 B.C.) reported that inscriptions on an Egyptian pyramid recorded the quantities of garlic consumed by the laborers. The Roman naturalist Pliny the Elder (A.D. 23–79) declared, "Garlic has powerful properties, and is of great benefit against changes of water and of residence." He recommended it to treat asthma, suppress coughs, and expel intestinal parasites, but noted some drawbacks (other than garlic breath): garlic dulled the sight, caused flatulence, injured the stomach if taken in excess, and caused thirst. In China, garlic was traditionally used for fevers, dysentery, and intestinal parasites. Its antibacterial activity was first recognized in an 1858 study by the French microbiologist Louis Pasteur.

Current Use: In the past 20 years garlic has been the subject of more than 2,500 credible scientific studies. Well-documented health benefits include reducing cholesterol and triglycerides in the blood (while increasing high-density lipoproteins, so-called good cholesterol), lowering blood pressure, improving circulation, and helping to prevent yeast infections, cancers, colds, and flu. Garlic has good antibacterial, antifungal, antiparasitic, antioxidant, anti-inflammatory, and immunostimulant properties. At least 9 epidemiological studies show that garlic significantly decreases the incidence of cancer, especially cancers of the gastrointestinal tract, among those who consume it regularly.

Nearly 3,000 patients have been involved in 18 clinical studies on the use of 600 to 900 mg of garlic powder to reduce blood lipids over a one- to four-month period. When taken together, the studies show an average reduction of 9 to 12 percent of total serum cholesterol, and a reduction of 13 percent of triglycerides, compared with placebo. It is considered a useful therapeutic tool for patients with milder forms of hyperlipidemia.

Another recent study found that eating the equivalent of one garlic clove (3 g) a day for several months had a significant blood-thinning effect.

When garlic is cut or crushed, it produces sulfur compounds, such as allicin, because a sulfur-containing amino acid, alliin, comes into contact with the enzyme allinase. Garlic has an extremely complex chemistry, with more than 160 compounds identified from its bulbs and essential oil.

If your food should be your medicine, garlic should be part of your diet.

Used For:
Chemoprevention • Lowering cholesterol

Preparations:
Fresh or dried cloves, capsules, "odorless" tablets, tinctures, aged garlic extracts.

Typical Dosages:
Capsules: Up to three 500–600 mg capsules a day, or follow manufacturer's or practitioner's recommendations. Look for products that deliver at least 5,000 micrograms of allicin daily.

Food: One or more fresh cloves a day. Eat raw or add to foods at the end of cooking to retain sulphur compounds.

Or follow manufacturer's or practitioner's recommendations.

Cautions:
Rare cases of allergic reactions to garlic have been reported. Some individuals experience heartburn or flatulence.

Gentian

Gentiana lutea

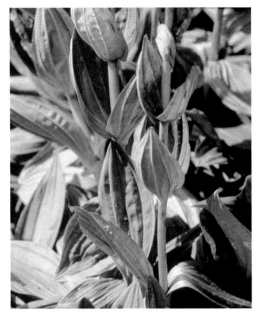

Sources: Gentian is the root of *G. lutea,* a member of the gentian family native to the mountains of central and southern Europe. The dried root of this yellow-flowered perennial is cultivated and wild-harvested.

Traditional Use: Gentian was mentioned in the works of the first-century Roman physicians Pliny and Dioscorides. Named after Gentius, an Illyrian king (180–167 B.C.), the herb has been used throughout history as a bitter digestive tonic. In 1865, a patent medicine containing gentian and licorice root was sold under the name "Tobacco Antidote," chewed to quell the desire for tobacco. This use seems to grow out of a reputation in medieval European folk medicine as an antidote to poisons. Gentian was an official drug of the *United States Pharmacopoeia* from 1820 to 1950.

> In 1865, a patent medicine containing gentian and licorice root was sold under the name "Tobacco Antidote," chewed to quell the desire for tobacco.

Current Use: Gentian root is widely used in European phytomedicines for gastrointestinal preparations, mostly combined with other herbs. The root is extremely bitter and stimulates the taste buds and brain reflexes to promote secretion of gastric juices and saliva. It is approved in a number of European countries as an appetite stimulant to treat anorexia, as a digestive tonic during convalescence, and as a treatment for dyspepsia, flatulence, and bloating. Results of modern pharmacological and clinical studies correlate well with traditional use.

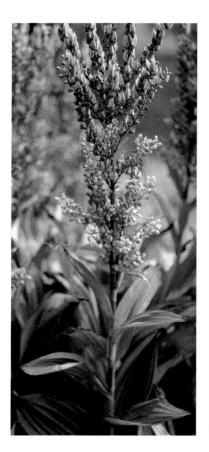

Used For:
Dyspepsia • Anorexia • Stimulating digestion

Preparations:
Dried root, cut and sifted or powdered; capsules; liquid extracts; tinctures.

Typical Dosages:
Tea: Steep 1/3 tsp dried root in 1 cup hot water for 10–15 minutes, or soak in cold water for 8 hours. Use 3 times a day before meals.
Tincture (1:5, 50% alcohol): 5–20 drops before meals.
Or follow manufacturer's or practitioner's recommendations.

Cautions:
The German health authorities state that use is contraindicated in the presence of stomach or duodenal ulcers. Some individuals may experience headaches from using gentian.

Ginger

Zingiber officinale

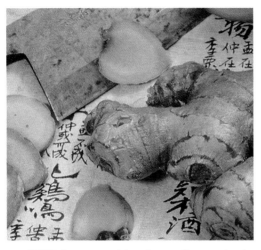

Source: Ginger is the dried or fresh root of a member of the ginger family native to the Old World tropics.

Traditional Use: Cultivated for millennia in both China and India, ginger reached the West at least 2,000 years ago. Most of the thousands of prescriptions in Traditional Chinese Medicine (TCM) are combinations of many herbs, and ginger is used in nearly half to mediate the effects of other ingredients, to stimulate the appetite, and to calm the stomach. In European herbal traditions, ginger is primarily used to stop nausea and quiet an stomach upset.

Current Use: Ginger is now recognized for treating stomach upset and easing symptoms of motion sickness. It is believed to reduce nausea by increasing digestive fluids and absorbing and neutralizing toxins and stomach acid. It increases bile secretion and tones the bowel.

It has been studied for its antibacterial, antifungal, pain-relieving, antiulcer, antitumor, and other properties. Six clinical studies have looked at ginger's potential to reduce motion sickness. Four European studies reported positive results, while two American studies gave negative findings. In an English study, thirty-six volunteers were given either ginger or a common anti-motion sickness drug. When blindfolded and subjected to a spinning chair, those who took ginger held out an average of 5.5 minutes, while those who took the conventional drug became ill after 3.5 minutes. Another study involved eighty naval cadets at sea. Those who took a placebo developed seasickness. Those who were given ginger root capsules had fewer cold sweats and less nausea. However, a 1988

NASA study that tested ginger in forty-two volunteers concluded it was ineffective in relieving motion sickness. Clearly, more studies are needed.

Ginger has been shown to reduce the stickiness of blood platelets and may thereby reduce the risk of atherosclerosis. Limited studies suggest ginger may reduce morning sickness and nausea after surgery. Both uses require a physician's supervision.

Other studies show that ginger may help reduce cholesterol and arterial plaque by transporting high-density lipoproteins to the liver where they can be metabolized and eliminated.

Used For:
Indigestion • Motion sickness • Nausea

Preparations:
Fresh or dried root, capsules, tablets, tinctures.

Typical Dosages:
Capsules: Up to eight 500–600 mg capsules a day, or follow manufacturer's or practitioner's recommendations.
Ground root: 1/2–1 tsp a day.
Tincture: 10–20 drops in water 3 times a day.
Or follow manufacturer's or practitioner's recommendations.

Cautions:
The German therapeutic monograph on ginger cautions against exceeding the recommend dosage. and warns patients with gallbladder disease not to take it. Pregnant women contemplating ginger use during morning sickness (short-term only) should avoid the root if gallbladder disease is present. Ginger has recognized blood-thinning qualities, but British research indicates that ginger is unlikely to cause adverse effects before or after surgery.

Ginkgo

Ginkgo biloba

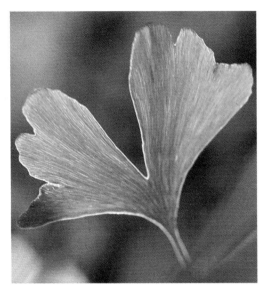

Sources: Ginkgo products come from the leaves of the only surviving member of the ginkgo family, a living fossil more than 200 million years old. Most commercial leaf production is from plantations in South Carolina, France, and China.

Traditional Use: Ginkgo leaf is a relatively new herbal medicine, used in China only since the fifteenth century. The leaves have traditionally been used for "benefitting the brain" and treating lung disorders, cough and asthma symptoms, and diarrhea. The leaf tea is applied externally to treat sores and remove freckles.

Current Use: Ginkgo is among the best-selling herbal medicines in Europe. Most research has focused on use of ginkgo to increase circulation to the extremities as well as the brain, especially in the elderly. Clinical use is supported by more than 400 scientific studies conducted since the late 1950s. Ginkgo extract has also been studied for the treatment of ringing in the ears (tinnitus), male impotence, degenerative nerve conditions such as multiple sclerosis, and other diseases. Ginkgo has demonstrated the potential to improve short-term memory, attention span, and mood in the early stages of Alzheimer disease by improving oxygen metabolism in the brain. The vast majority of studies have involved an extract called EGb-761.

A 1996 controlled study looked at the effect of a ginkgo-leaf extract in the treatment of outpatients with dementia associated with Alzheimer. Twenty-eight percent of patients in the treatment group responded positively to the ginkgo leaf extract, compared with 10 percent in the placebo group.

The first large-scale American clinical study on ginkgo was published in 1997 in the *Journal of the American Medical Association.* Focusing on ginkgo's effect on improving the short-term memory of early diagnosed Alzheimer disease, the researchers concluded that the herb is safe and stabilizing, and that, in a significant number of patients, it improves cognitive performance and social functioning.

Ginkgo's effects have been attributed to flavone glycosides and ginkgolides, unique compounds that inhibit platelet-activating factor involved in the development of inflammatory, cardiovascular, and respiratory disorders. Ginkgolides' activity helps explain the herb's broad-spectrum biological effects.

One reason for this conclusion is ginkgo's strong antioxidant activity. By "scavenging" free radicals, ginkgo directs antioxidant effects to the brain, central nervous system, and cardiovascular system. This mechanism makes it promising in the treatment of age-related declines of brain function.

Used For:
Age-related memory loss • Tinnitus • Improving microcirculation

Preparations:
Dried leaf, tea. Highly concentrated leaf extract, standardized to 24% flavone glycosides and further calibrated for 6% ginkgolides, with potentially toxic ginkgolic acid removed.

Typical Dosage:
Capsules: 3 capsules containing at least 40 mg of standardized extract a day, or follow manufacturer's or practitioner's recommendations. Ginkgo must be used for 6–8 weeks before results are evident.

Cautions:
Rare cases of gastrointestinal upset, headaches, or skin allergies have been reported. In any such case, use of ginkgo should be discontinued.

Ginseng
Panax quinquefolius, P. ginseng

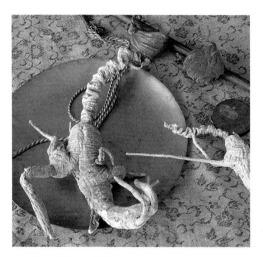

Sources: Ginseng is the root of two different herbs from opposite sides of the world, American ginseng (*Panax quinquefolius*) and Asian ginseng (*P. ginseng*). American ginseng grows in eastern North America and is wild-harvested. Asian ginseng, which includes both Korean and Chinese ginseng, is cultivated in China, Korea, and Japan.

Traditional Use: According to the Harvard University botanist Shiu Ying Hu, the earliest mention of ginseng is in the 2,000-year-old herbal of Shen Nong, which reports ginseng's use for repairing the five viscera, quieting the spirit, curbing the emotions, stopping agitation, removing noxious influences, brightening the eyes, enlightening the mind, and increasing wisdom. Continuous use leads one to "longevity with light weight." Ginseng use has changed little in 2,000 years.

Current Use: In the last thirty years, Asian ginseng (but not American ginseng) has been extensively studied. Like eleuthero, ginseng is an adaptogen. At least seven European clinical studies have shown that standardized extracts decrease reaction time to visual and auditory stimuli; increase respiratory performance, alertness, power of concentration, and grasp of abstract concepts; and improve visual and motor coordination. Sometimes conflicting results indicate the need for further clinical studies, especially on products with well-defined levels of active compounds.

A controlled study in France evaluated complaints of patients suffering from "functional fatigue," such as being worn out, tired, empty-feeling, etc. Results showed that patients receiving the ginseng product experienced significant improvement in reducing fatigue, anxiety, and poor concentration compared with patients who received the placebo.

Recent studies have focused on antiviral and metabolic effects, antioxidant activity, and effects on nervous and reproductive systems.

Ginseng is also a nonspecific immunostimulant similar to echinacea. There are more than eighteen active chemicals called ginsenosides in Asian ginseng. American and Asian ginsengs contain some of the same as well as some different ginsenosides, which explains their different actions as expressed in Traditional Chinese Medicine. Mild American ginseng helps to reduce the heat of the respiratory and digestive systems, whereas the stronger Asian ginseng is a heat-raising tonic for the blood and circulatory systems.

In Germany, Asian ginseng products may be labeled as tonics to treat fatigue, reduced work capacity, lack of concentration, and convalescence.

Used For:
Convalescence • Fatigue • Improving concentration and well-being

Preparations:
Asian: dried root ("white"), steamed root ("red"); capsules, extracts, tablets, tinctures, teas. Some products are standardized to 4–7% ginsenosides. *American:* dried root, whole or powdered; capsules, tinctures.

Typical Dosage:
Capsules: Up to four 500–600 mg capsules a day. For standardized products, 100 mg 1 or 2 times a day is generally recommended. Or follow manufacturer's or practitioner's recommendations.

Cautions:
Use at normal dosage levels is generally not associated with side effects; however, some persons have experienced over-stimulation or gastrointestinal upset; some women have reported breast tenderness or menstrual problems following long-term use. If you have high blood pressure, use ginseng with caution. Avoid ginseng during pregnancy.

Goldenseal

Hydrastis canadensis

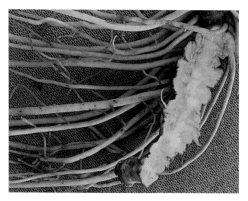

Source: Goldenseal is the root and rhizome of a member of the buttercup family that grows in rich woods from Vermont to Georgia, west to Alabama and Arkansas, and north to eastern Iowa and Minnesota. Wild-harvested material is becoming increasingly scarce (and high-priced), but many start-up goldenseal cultivation projects were initiated in the 1990s.

Traditional Use: The Cherokee used goldenseal roots to treat inflammations and drank a root tea to improve appetite and treat dyspepsia. The Iroquois used goldenseal for liver disorders, fever, sour stomach, and diarrhea.

Goldenseal was listed among the official remedies in the first revision (1830) of the New York edition of the *United States Pharmacopoeia*. It was dropped in 1840, then listed again from 1860 to 1926. The root was used primarily for inflammations of the mucous membranes.

Current Use: Goldenseal is one of the more popular American herbs. It is used as an antiseptic, to stop bleeding, and as a tonic and anti-inflammatory for the mucous membranes. Components derived from the root have been used in eyewashes.

Goldenseal's major effects are attributed to the alkaloids hydrastine and berberine. In animal experiments, hydrastine lowers blood pressure; berberine, which gives goldenseal its yellow color and bitter taste, stimulates digestion and the secretion of bile, lowers blood pressure, reduces muscle spasms, and inhibits growth of bacteria.

A recent study on the effect of isolated chemicals from goldenseal in reducing muscle contractions showed that rather than being dependent upon the effects of a single chemical component, a synergistic action of several compounds produces the effects, while an additional compound, hydrastine, helps to moderate that effect. This shows that the sum of the chemical parts of this medicinal plant is greater than its individual components. Herbal medicine is based on using whole plant parts rather than their single isolated chemical components.

One modern folk use of goldenseal, based on the plot of a 1900 novel by the pharmacist John Uri Lloyd, *Stringtown on the Pike,* is ingesting the herb in an attempt to mask the presence of illicit drugs in the urine. Although there is no scientific evidence to support this practice, some laboratories now test for goldenseal in urinalysis. Still widely used, goldenseal is a plant in need of new research.

Used For:
Inflammation of mucous membrane • Fighting infection

Preparations:
Dried root, whole or powdered; leaf; capsules, extracts, ointments, salves, tablets, tinctures.

Typical Dosages:
Capsules: Up to six 500–600 mg capsules a day, or follow manufacturer's or practitioner's recommendations.
Tincture (1:5, 70% alcohol): 20–50 drops.
Or follow manufacturer's or practitioner's recommendations.

Cautions:
Applications of fresh goldenseal may cause ulcerations of the skin; however, reports of this reaction relate to homeopathic remedies of the mid-nineteenth century that added jimsonweed and zinc oxide to goldenseal. No recent reports of toxicity occur in the literature. Several books warn pregnant and nursing women and people with heart problems to use goldenseal cautiously, presumably because of the lack of toxicity studies. While it has not been documented scientifically, goldenseal may disrupt intestinal flora; some herbalists recommend taking acidophilus with goldenseal.

Gotu Kola

Centella asiatica (formerly *Hydrocotyle asiatica*)

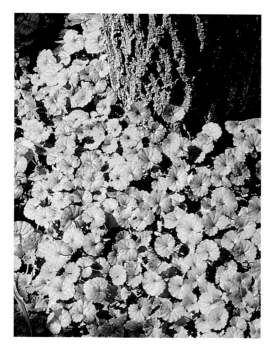

Source: Gotu kola is a low-growing herb in the parsley family native to tropical Asia, where it is grown commercially. It also grows in Hawaii and other tropical regions.

Traditional Use: In India, the ancient tradition of Ayurveda regards gotu kola as an important rejuvenating herb, especially for nerve and brain cells. It is prescribed to increase intelligence, longevity, and memory while retarding senility and aging. A leaf tea is used as a wash for skin diseases, inflammation, and swelling. In Chinese folk medicine, the leaf tea is used internally for colds and lung and urinary tract infections, and externally for snakebite, injuries, and shingles.

Current Use: The notion that gotu kola promotes intelligence has led to a number of studies of its effect on the central nervous system. Preliminary results show that it can be beneficial in improving memory and may also help overcome stress and fatigue.

Two older Indian studies report that it helps improve intelligence, general mental abilities, and behavior in mentally retarded children. In a subsequent study, rats given an extract of fresh gotu kola leaves for two weeks scored three to sixty times better than untreated rats in tests of learning and memory.

Other experiments indicate that gotu kola acts as a mild depressant on the central nervous system. Topically, it relieves inflammation and helps rebuild damaged skin tissue. In one clinical study of a topical preparation, thirteen of twenty patients with poorly healing wounds experienced complete, accelerated healing.

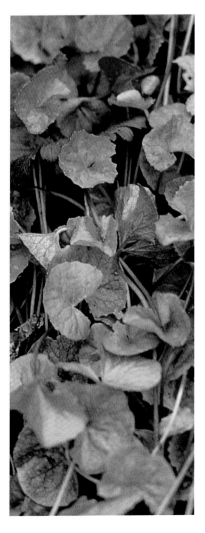

Used For:
Improving memory • Stress reduction

Preparations:
Dried herb, cut and sifted or powdered; capsules; tablets; tinctures; teas. In other countries, standardized to asiaticoside.

Typical Dosages:
Capsules: Up to eight 400–500 mg capsules a day.
Tea: Steep 1 tsp dried herb in 1 cup of hot water for 10–15 minutes.
Tincture (1:5, 50% alcohol): 20–40 drops up to 2 times a day.
Or follow manufacturer's or practitioner's recommendations.

Cautions:
None noted.

Grapeseed
Vitis vinifera

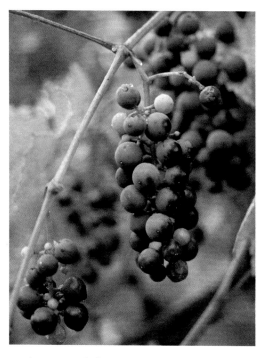

Sources: The seed of *Vitis vinifera,* a member of the grape vine family, is now emerging as an important new ingredient in dietary supplements. While grapes have long provided the world with food and drink, it is only in recent years that the seeds have found a commercial use.

Traditional Use: Grapes have been food since before recorded history; their use for wine dates back at least 4,500 years to ancient Egypt. All parts of the plant have been used for medicinal purposes: the leaves as an astringent for treating everything from diarrhea to varicose veins; the juice of unripe fruits for sore throat; raisins for sore throats, coughs, and cooling. The pharmacology of wine dates to the first sip. Now we know that red wine in particular has positive antioxidant health benefits.

> **Grapeseed's strong antioxidant, anti-mutagenic action may serve to protect against disease development.**

Current Use: Grapeseed's strong antioxidant, antimutagenic action may serve to protect against disease development. Procyanidins in grapeseed reduce altered capillary permeability. This effect has proven useful in standardized products for microcirculatory disorders, such as diseases related to problems in capillary resistance and permeability of cells in the skin, as well as circulatory problems. One study found that as little as a single, 150-mg dose of procyanidins helps to increase venous tone in patients with widespread varicose veins. In the treatment of eye conditions, procyanidins promote resistance to glare and improvement of night vision. Grapeseed's antioxidant, anti-inflammatory activity helps slow the aging process in skin and protects against radiation effects.

Used For:
Varicose veins • Circulatory problems • Poor vision • Antioxidant

Preparations:
Extract. The active chemical is oligomeric procyanidins (OPC).

Typical Dosage:
Extract: 150 mg of procyanidins a day. Follow manufacturer's instructions.

Cautions:
None noted.

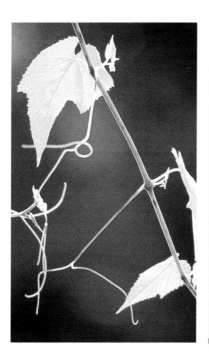

Hawthorn

Crataegus spp.

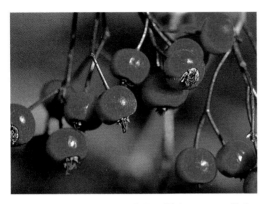

Sources: Hawthorn is the fruit, or the flowers and leaves combined, of several of the more than 100 species of *Crataegus,* a genus of the rose family found in North America, Europe, and east Asia. In Europe, English hawthorn, *C. laevigata,* and oneseed hawthorn, *C. monogyna,* are used. In Chinese medicine, *C. pinnatifida* is used.

Traditional Use: If closely related plants are used by cultures on opposite sides of the globe, a scientific basis for that use is likely. Such is the case with hawthorn, which has been used in European, Chinese, and American traditions alike to treat heart ailments. Asian and European herbal traditions have used hawthorn in long-term prescriptions for hypertension related to cardiac weakness, arteriosclerosis, and angina pectoris.

Hawthorn is notably absent from medical works and herbals of early-nineteenth-century America and Europe. It came to the attention of the medical profession in the 1890s by means of a single reference in a medical journal. By the early twentieth century, it was a mainstay of heart disease treatment. Still widely used in Europe and Asia, it is less frequently recommended in America.

Current Use: Medical practitioners in Europe and China use hawthorn to treat early stages of congestive heart failure characterized by diminished cardiac function, a sensation of pressure or anxiety in the heart area, age-related heart disorders which do not require digitalis, and mild arrhythmias. Numerous pharmacological and clinical studies have shown that hawthorn fruit or berry extract improves blood flow to and from the heart by strengthening its contractions. Hawthorn flower and leaf extracts improve circulation to the extremities by reducing resistance in the arteries. Hawthorn preparations do not produce immediate effects; rather, they must be used over a period of at least four to eight weeks to achieve therapeutic benefits.

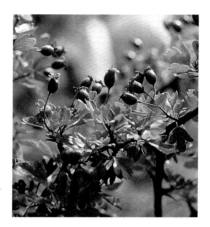

Experiments in China have shown that preparations of hawthorn fruit lower blood pressure and serum cholesterol levels, and are therefore useful in the prevention and treatment of arteriosclerosis.

Used For:
Angina pectoris • Early stages of congestive heart failure • Coronary insufficiency

Preparations:
Dried berries, leaves, flowers. Most research has been done on flowers and leaves. Standardized in Europe to oligomeric procyanidins and flavonoids.

Typical Dosages:
Capsules (non-standardized): Up to nine 500–600 mg capsules a day.
Tea: Steep 1 tsp of dried berries in a cup of hot water for 10–15 minutes.
Tincture (1:5, 60% alcohol): 10–30 drops up to 3 times a day.
Or follow manufacturer's or practitioner's recommendations.

Cautions:
No side effects or contraindications are known for hawthorn. Any heart condition, however, is serious and should receive the attention of qualified health-care practitioners. Heart disease is the number-one killer in America; it should not be self-diagnosed or self-treated.

Hops

Humulus lupulus

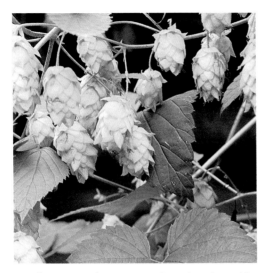

Source: Hops are the fruiting bodies or strobiles of a member of the cannabis family native to Europe, Asia, and North America. Hops are widely grown in the Pacific Northwest, Germany, and the Czech Republic, and are used primarily for flavoring beer.

Traditional Use: Traditionally, hops have been considered soothing to the stomach, an appetite stimulant (due to the bitter taste), slightly sedative, a sleep aid, and diuretic. A popular way of using hops as a sleep aid was to stuff a pillow with the fruiting bodies, moistening them slightly before bed to prevent them from rustling and keeping an insomniac awake! A hops poultice was used to relieve pain of rheumatic joints and a tea was taken to relieve muscle spasms and soothe the nerves.

Current Use: In European phytomedicine, hops preparations are used to relieve mood disturbances, such as unrest and anxiety, and for sleep disturbances. Hops are also prescribed for nervous tension, excitability, restlessness and lack of sleep, and to stimulate appetite. Laboratory studies show that hops have a wide range of biological activity. Bitter acids in the fruits are antibacterial. Fruit extracts strongly reduce smooth-muscle spasms. Studies have both confirmed and disputed hops' sedative and estrogenic activities.

Use of hops as a sedative is a relatively recent development. A condition called hop-picker fatigue was reported in which hops pickers were observed to become tired easily, perhaps because of contact with the resin or inhaling the essential oil. Sedative action has been attributed to a volatile compound in hops that would be present in hops pillows (though absent from extracts), which provides a rational basis for the traditional use of hops-filled pillows to aid sleep. In Germany it is approved for discomfort from restlessness or anxiety and sleep disturbances.

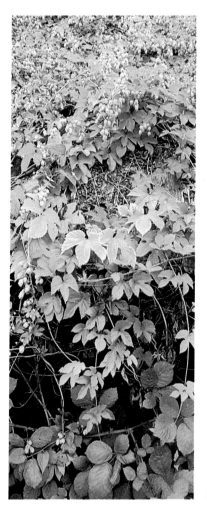

Used For:
Anxiety • Insomnia • Lack of appetite

Preparations:
Dried strobiles; capsules, tablets, tinctures, tea. Also used in combination products with valerian, passionflower, and skullcap.

Typical Dosages:
Tea: Steep 1 heaping tsp whole dried hops in 1 cup hot water for 10–15 minutes. Take before bedtime.
Tincture: 10–40 drops 3 times a day.
Or follow manufacturer's or practitioner's recommendations.

Cautions:
No side effects, contraindications, or adverse drug interactions from the use of hops are generally reported, though some individuals have experienced a rare allergic reaction or contact dermatitis from the pollen or the yellow powder-like crystals in the fruits.

Horehound

Marrubium vulgare

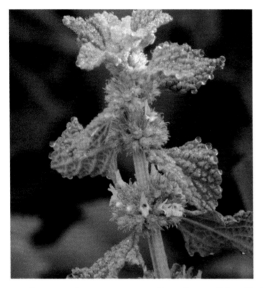

Sources: Horehound is the whole herb of a fuzzy gray perennial member of the mint family found in waste places throughout much of Europe and naturalized in North America and elsewhere. The whole dried herb, harvested while in flower, is used.

Traditional Use: Horehound has been an important European folk medicine since early times. Unlike most mints, which have a pleasant aroma, horehound has little aroma and a bitter flavor. Horehound has been used as a domestic remedy for coughs and congestion, tea to stimulate bile, and for the treatment of liver conditions. It was an official remedy of the *United States Pharmacopoeia* from 1820 to 1900.

> This herb's traditional use as a cough suppressant, expectorant, and bitter digestive tonic has stood the test of time.

Current Use: In modern phytomedicine, horehound and its preparations are used as an appetite stimulant (for anorexia) and a feeling of fullness in the stomach with flatulence, as well as catarrhs of the upper respiratory tract. Pharmacological studies have also shown that it stimulates bile production. It is approved for the above uses in Germany and a number of other European countries. The herb was an approved over-the-counter drug ingredient in the United States until 1989, when it was banned because of lack of data on effectiveness and safety. (None was submitted.) This herb's traditional use as a cough suppressant, expectorant, and bitter digestive tonic has stood the test of time. More research needs to be done to bring it back into modern acceptance.

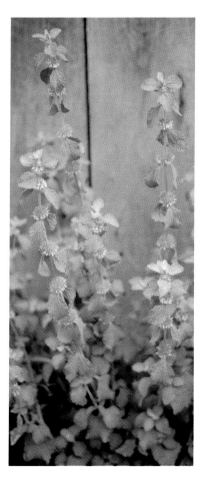

Used For:
Anorexia • Coughs and catarrhs • Digestion

Preparations:
Dried herb, cut and sifted; extract (used to flavor cough drops and candies).

Typical Dosages:
Lozenges: Follow manufacturer's instructions.
Tea: Steep 2–3 tsp dried herb in 1 cup hot water for 10–15 minutes. Use 2 or 3 times a day.

Cautions:
No side effects, contraindications, or interactions with other drugs are known.

Horse Chestnut

Aesculus hippocastanum

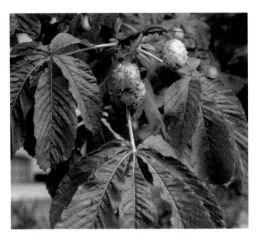

Sources: Horse chestnut consists of preparations made from the bark, seeds, and leaves of this large tree, native to central Asia and introduced into western Europe around 1576. Horse chestnut is commonly grown as a shade tree in the United States. Much of the modern medicinal supply is produced in Poland. At least six *Aesculus* species and several hybrids are native to North America.

Traditional Use: Capitalizing on the astringent effects of tannin, the bark has been used as a folk medicine for the treatment of diarrhea and hemorrhoids. A tea of the leaves sweetened with honey has been used as a cough remedy and a treatment for arthritis and rheumatism. Poisonous qualities attributed to the seeds stem from use by Native Americans who ground or decocted the seeds to stupefy fish.

Current Use: Horse chestnut extracts (primarily from the seeds) are used in modern phytomedicine to help improve vascular resistance to damage, reduce capillary-wall permeability, and absorb damaging UV radiation. Such products contain a compound called aescin (or escin) that diminishes the number or diameter of tiny openings in capillary walls, helping to "seal" the outflow of fluid into surrounding tissue. This unique mechanism of action makes it very useful for the topical treatment of bruises, sprains and contusions. In addition, standardized oral dosage forms have been the subject of a number of controlled clinical studies which show them to be valuable in aiding chronic venous insufficiency, reducing leg edema, improving vascular tone, and mitigating subjective symptoms such as a feeling of heaviness in the legs, night-time calf muscle spasms, itching, and swelling. It is the single most widely prescribed remedy in Germany for edema with venous insufficiency. Injectable forms are used in the treatment of severe head trauma and to reduce postoperative swelling in surgery.

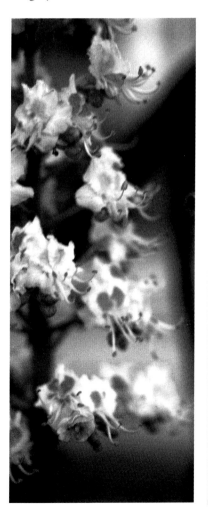

Used For:
Chronic venous insufficiency • Bruises • Sprains • Edema

Preparations:
Capsules, tablets, standardized products.

Typical Dosage:
Extract: 30–150 mg a day.
Or follow manufacturer's or practitioner's recommendations.

Cautions:
In rare instances, internal use may cause stomach upset. Occasional nausea and itching have also been reported. In Europe, controlled-release forms are available that reduce the chance of stomach upset. No contraindications or interactions with other drugs are known. The crude herb (including bark, leaves, or seeds) could be potentially toxic. Only standardized, manufactured preparations can be recommended for use.

Horsetail

Equisetum spp.

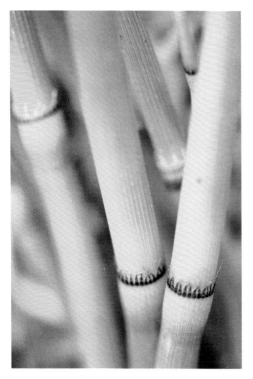

Sources: Horsetails, also known as shavegrass and scouring rush, are species of a primitive nonflowering plant group in the genus *Equisetum*. The most commonly used species are *E. hyemale* (often called scouring rush), and *E. arvense* (field horsetail). Both occur throughout the Northern Hemisphere. Use of certain horsetails, such as *E. palustre*, which contains a toxic alkaloid, palustrine, should be avoided. Most of the supply comes from Europe or China, though horsetail is common in North America as well.

Traditional Use: Horsetails have traditionally been used as herbal diuretics. They have a very high silica content, which also accounts for their traditional use of the stems as a natural scouring pad or even sandpaper. In tea, horsetail has been used as a folk remedy to treat bloody urine, gout, stomach problems, and gonorrhea. Externally, it has been poulticed to stop bleeding and to treat rheumatism, fractures, and sprains.

Current Use: Studies on the chemistry, pharmacology, and clinical implications of horsetail preparations have been conducted in Europe over the last twenty years. The silica content is up to 15 percent, consisting of silicic acids and silicates. They are up to 80 percent water-soluble, depending upon processing methods used.

Horsetail is recognized for its mild diuretic qualities; flavonoids are thought to be responsible for this action. An advantage it may have over other herb diuretics is that horsetail produces a diuretic effect without increasing the excretion of electrolytes. Human clinical studies are generally absent from the literature. However, it is approved in Germany as a diuretic for edema, and bacterial-induced inflammatory conditions of the urinary tract.

Topically, horsetail has been shown to have a styptic effect, and strengthens and regenerates connective tissue (thought to be due to the silica content). In Germany, it is approved for external use to help treat poorly healing wounds.

Used For:
Diuresis • Healing wounds

Preparations:
Whole herb, cut and sifted or powdered; capsules; tablets; tinctures; combination products.

Typical Dosages:
Capsules: Up to six 400–500 mg capsules a day.
Tea: Steep 2 tsp in 1 cup of hot water for 10–15 minutes. Use up to 6 times a day.
Tincture: 15–30 drops 3 times a day.
Wash (external): Soak 10 tsp dried herb in cold water for 10–12 hours and apply as needed.
Or follow manufacturer's or practitioner's recommendations.

Cautions:
Proper identification of species is important since some *Equisetums* are classified as poisonous plants. There is evidence that *E. arvense* contains an enzyme that interferes with thiamin metabolism. Children, people with heart or kidney disease, and pregnant or nursing women should not use horsetail. No one should use it long term because clear data on toxicity is lacking.

Hyssop

Hyssopus officinalis

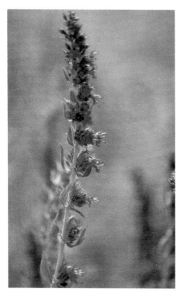

Sources: Hyssop is a perennial member of the mint family native to southern, south-central, and eastern Europe. In America, it is commonly grown in herb gardens and has occasionally escaped. Most of the commercial supply comes from Europe. The above-ground parts, harvested when in flower, are used.

Traditional Use: One of the best known botanical lines in the Bible is Psalms 51:7: "Purge me with *Hyssop*, and I shall be clean." But if we look at a long line of opinions by botanical biblical scholars, perhaps the line should instead read, "Purge me with capers. . . ." The "hyssop" of the Bible probably does not refer to *H. officinalis.*

In European folk traditions, hyssop has been used in combination with horehound to treat lung ailments associated with coughs and colds, asthma, and bronchitis. Hyssop tea is gargled for sore throats. Externally, the herb has been used to treat rheumatism, muscle aches, wounds, and sprains. In the eighteenth edition of *King's American Dispensatory*, Harvey Wickes Felter and John Uri Lloyd highlight this use: "The leaves, applied to bruises, speedily relieve the pain, and disperse every spot or mark from the parts affected." Now there's a research lead for an enterprising graduate student.

Current Use: Never recognized as an important herb by the medical profession, hyssop deserves a closer look. Extracts of hyssop have demonstrated anti-inflammatory activity and antiviral effects against herpes. Hyssop also has mild antioxidant activity. Hyssop extracts, presumably because of known antiviral activity, have been the subject of a couple of preliminary studies on anti-HIV activity.

In 1990 researchers reported that hyssop extract inhibited replication of human immunodeficiency virus. The research group identified caffeic acid in the extracts, along with unspecified tannins, and suggested that there may be a third group of high molecular-weight compounds with anti-HIV activity.

In 1995 another research group identified a polysaccharide that inhibited the SF strain of HIV-1, helping to prevent replication of the virus. The compound was also found not to have any significant direct toxic effect on the function of lymphocytes and specific T-cell counts. What these two studies indicate is that compounds in the plant seem to have an antiviral effect in laboratory test systems. It does not mean that hyssop will be found useful as a treatment for humans! More research is necessary.

Hyssop also contains antioxidant components associated with antiviral and anti-inflammatory activity. In European herbal traditions, the herb is most valued as a carminative and expectorant. Look for research to unlock more uses in the future.

Used For:
Folk remedy for colds and flu • Reducing gas in the digestive system

Preparations:
Dried herb, cut and sifted or powdered; capsules, tinctures, combination products.

Typical Dosages:
Capsules: Up to six 400–500 mg capsules a day.
Tea: Steep 1 tsp dried herb in 1 cup hot water for 10–15 minutes.
Tinctures: 10 to 40 drops up to 4 times a day.
Or follow manufacturer's or practitioner's recommendations.

Cautions:
None is noted for the dried herb. Essential oil of hyssop has been associated with at least three cases of poisoning, with as little as 2 to 3 drops producing toxicity in children; as little as 10 drops have caused spasms in adults. The herb is the subject of a negative regulatory monograph in Germany. Since traditional uses are unsubstantiated, medicinal claims are not allowed.

Juniper
Juniperus communis

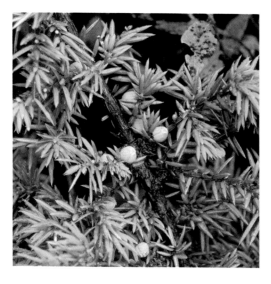

Sources: Juniper "berries" (technically cones) are harvested from the evergreen *Juniperus communis,* a common low-growing shrub of eastern North America. In Europe, the very same species takes on a different habit, growing into a taller shrub shaped like a Christmas tree. Most of the commercial supply comes from eastern and northern Europe.

Traditional Use: Juniper berries are best known for the characteristic flavoring of gin. The berries have been traditionally used in Europe to aid digestion, usually as tea, and applied externally to treat rheumatism, arthritis, and snakebite.

In Germany, juniper berries are approved for use in the treatment of dyspeptic complaints and as an appetite stimulant.

Current Use: Juniper is most widely used as an herbal diuretic and urinary antiseptic. Anti-inflammatory and antispasmodic activity has been confirmed. While often used as a diuretic, it can irritate the bladder and kidneys. In Germany, it is approved for use in the treatment of dyspeptic complaints and as an appetite stimulant. Despite the fact it is approved for use, little clinical research has been published.

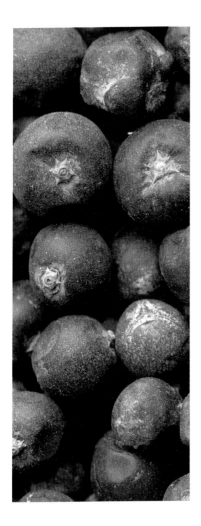

Used For:
Dyspeptic complaints •
Diuresis

Preparations:
Whole dried berries, cut and sifted or powdered; capsules, tablets, tinctures.

Typical Dosages:
Berries: 1 tsp crushed berries a day.
Capsules: Up to six 400–500 mg capsules a day.
Tincture: 15–30 drops 3 times a day.
Or follow manufacturer's or practitioner's recommendations.

Cautions:
German health authorities warn that use of juniper berries is contraindicated in pregnancy and inflammatory kidney diseases. In any case, use is limited to four weeks because long-term use or overdose can lead to kidney damage. Diabetics are warned that ingesting juniper berries can raise glucose levels.

Kava-kava

Piper methysticum

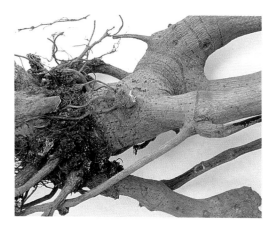

Source: Kava-kava, or kava as it is also known, is the massive root or leaf of a highly variable sprawling shrub in the pepper family, found throughout the South Pacific islands from Hawaii to New Guinea. The plant has been cultivated for so many centuries that its exact origin is unclear. Like garlic, kava in its present form has evolved over thousands of years of cultivation. Now the kava craze is upon the United States. The only problem is, at this writing, that the demand far outstrips the limited supply from the South Pacific.

Traditional Use: Polynesians have used a thick brew of the fresh or dried kava root as their main beverage for centuries. A similar beverage, prepared from ground roots, is often imbibed in social or ceremonial settings. The cultural role of kava in Pacific societies has been compared to that of wine in southern Europe. A decoction of the rootstock has reportedly been used for the treatment of gonorrhea, chronic cystitis and other urinary infections, menstrual problems, migraine headache, insomnia, and other conditions.

The first herb products made from kava appeared in Europe in the 1860s. By the 1890s, kava extracts were available in German herb shops. The first pharmaceutical preparation, a tincture used as a mild sedative and to lower blood pressure, became available in Germany thirty years later.

Current Use: In Germany the rootstock and its preparations are allowed to be labeled for conditions of nervous anxiety, stress, and unrest. In Europe, for the treatment of irritable bladder syndrome, kava extracts are often combined with pumpkin seed for its diuretic effect.

Kava compounds called kavalactones have pain-relieving effects comparable to aspirin. One kavalactone produces a numbing effect in the mouth upon chewing the root or drinking kava preparations. Kavalactones have been shown to relax muscles by affecting muscular contractility rather than by blocking neurotransmitter signals in nerves.

At least seven controlled clinical studies have confirmed the use of kava for anxiety, tension, and excitedness. Since the conventional drugs used to treat anxiety—tranquilizers, neuroleptics, and antidepressants—may carry the risk of addiction or severe side effects, European practitioners often turn to kava for proven effectiveness and few side effects.

Used For:
Anxiety • Insomnia • Stress

Preparations:
Dried root, capsules, tablets, tinctures.

Typical Dosages:
Capsules: Up to six 400–500 mg capsules a day.
Tincture: 15–30 drops in water up to 3 times a day.
Or follow manufacturer's or practitioner's recommendations.

Cautions:
The German health authorities warn that kava should not be used during pregnancy, lactation, or depression. Because of its apparent sedative action, it should not be taken with alcohol or when operating machinery or vehicles. No side effects are associated with small amounts of kava. In the copious amounts consumed on South Sea islands, side effects of long-term use include temporary yellow discoloration of the skin, hair, and nails; rare allergic skin reactions; and vision disturbances. Excessive use has also caused itching and sores. In some popular Western articles and books, kava has been described as a "hypnotic," but contrary to the wishful thinking of some promoters, it is neither hallucinogenic nor stupefying, nor does it produce any physical addiction.

Kudzu

Pueraria montana

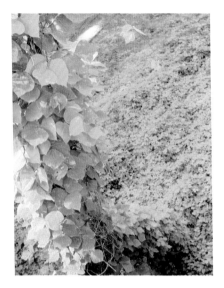

Sources: Kudzu as found on the market is the dried root of *Pueraria montana* (also designated *P. lobata* and *P. montana* var. *lobata* in recent literature), a fast-growing herbaceous vine in the pea family native to Asia. Seventeen species of *Pueraria* are recognized, yet only *P. montana* is found in North America, as a pernicious, even voracious weed, covering millions of acres in the southeastern United States. It was introduced as an erosion control and economically useful plant in the late nineteenth century. The root is the primary plant part used in herbal traditions.

Traditional Use: Kudzu has many uses. Before sweet potatoes were introduced to southeast Asia, kudzu root, which contains up to 27 percent starch, was widely used as a staple food. It has been valued for fiber, livestock silage, and many medicinal uses. In Japan, the plant's benefits date to A.D. 600. The huge root, often larger than a man, produces a processed starch used as a colloidal thickener. The root is also used as a jelling agent and for making noodles and texturing manufactured food goods. In China, kudzu is used to treat diarrhea and dysentery and to bring out skin eruptions when a disease is manifest beneath the skin and has yet to "reach the surface." The leaves, flowers, and seeds are also used in Asian traditions.

Current Use: Tablets manufactured from the root are used in modern China to treat angina pectoris and early symptoms of deafness. Experimentally the isoflavones in the root reduce blood pressure and venous obstructions. Extracts have been shown to improve symptoms associated with high blood pressure such as headache, vertigo, stiff neck, and ringing in the ears. Antioxidant components of kudzu root have been compared with vitamin E in preventing the oxidation of linoleic acid. An extract of the root has been shown to have 100 times the antioxidant activity of vitamin E. Puerarin has been identified as the active component.

A widely publicized 1993 study stimulated current interest in kudzu as a possible method for controlling the urge to drink. In this study daily doses of kudzu isoflavones were found to suppress the free choice of ethanol in Syrian Golden hamsters. The authors concluded that kudzu-root extracts may offer therapeutic choices in the treatment of alcohol abuse. This study confirmed traditional use of the application of the root (as well as the flowers) for the treatment of patients under the influence of alcohol.

Based on its potential use for controlling alcohol abuse, and the fact that it has been widely used as a folk medicine in India, researchers at Jiwaji University in India have determined that kudzu extract helps stimulate regeneration of the liver and makes the liver more resistant to damage from toxins.

Used For:
Angina pectoris • Reducing desire for alcohol

Preparations:
Dried herb, root, starch.

Typical Dosages:
Capsules: Up to six 150 mg capsules a day, or follow manufacturer's or practitioner's recommendations.
Tea: Steep 1 tsp powdered root in 1 cup hot water for 10–15 minutes. Use up to 3 times a day.
Tincture: 20–40 drops up to 5 times a day.
Or follow manufacturer's or practitioner's recommendations.

Cautions: None noted, except don't plant kudzu in your yard. If you do, mulch with cement blocks to control. Ingestion of kudzu is considered safe, without associated toxicity.

Lemon Balm

Melissa officinalis

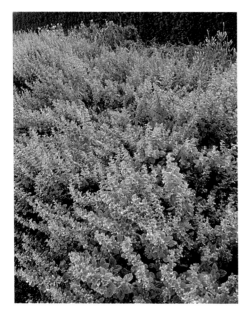

Source: Lemon balm is the leaf of a perennial herb in the mint family native to the Mediterranean region, western Asia, southwestern Siberia, and northern Africa. It is widely naturalized in North America and elsewhere.

Traditional Use: Lemon balm's history dates back at least 2,000 years. It has been used to reduce fevers, induce sweating, calm the digestive tract, treat colds, and relieve spasms related to cramps and headaches. In medieval Europe, the tea was valued for disorders of the nervous system. It has long been a popular folk remedy for insomnia. Lemon balm was official in the *United States Pharmacopoeia* from 1840 to 1890.

Current Use: Lemon balm has been shown to be sedative, to relieve spasms, and inhibit the growth of fungi and bacteria. The German government allows preparations of lemon balm to be labeled for difficulty in falling asleep due to nervous conditions and for spasms of the digestive tract.

Laboratory experiments have shown activity against viruses, including mumps and herpes. A lemon-balm cream is sold in Germany for cold sores and conditions related to *Herpes simplex.* In a clinical study of 115 patients with herpes, a cream containing 1 percent dried lemon-balm extract was applied by the patients as needed five times daily for up to fourteen days. In 96 percent of the patients, lesions were healed by day eight of the treatment, in 87 percent by day six, and in 60 percent by day four. Unassisted healing usually takes ten to fourteen days. A subsequent controlled study compared the effectiveness of the same cream with a placebo. Both physicians and patients judged the lemon balm cream superior to the placebo, but it was found that treatment must be started very early in the infection, since accelerated healing was most pronounced in the first two days. Despite these findings, the German regulatory monograph for lemon balm does not mention use for treating herpes.

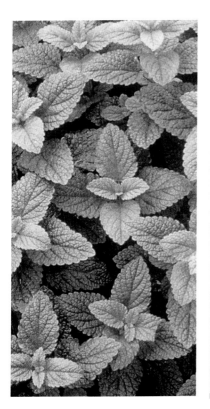

Used For:
Digestive gas • Herpes sores • Insomnia

Preparations:
Dried leaf, capsules, creams.

Typical Dosages:
Capsules: Up to nine 300–400 mg capsules a day.
Cream: Apply as directed at early stages of cold sores and genital herpes (not approved in the United States).
Tea: Steep 1½–4 tsp dried herb in 1 cup hot water for 10–15 minutes.
Or follow manufacturer's or practitioner's recommendations.

Cautions:
None noted.

Lemon Grass

Cymbopogon citratus

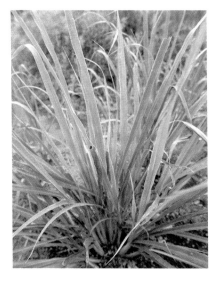

Sources: Lemon grass is a member of the grass family found in tropical regions throughout the world. Grown commercially, this perennial has evolved largely through human cultivation and rarely flowers. The dried leaves and the essential oil distilled from the leaves are widely available as flavorings in the United States.

Traditional Use: Lemon grass is a sleeper in the American market, not because it is traditionally used as a sleep aid, but because much of the American herb market is driven by European research, and lemon grass is rarely used in Europe except as a flavoring. However, in tropical Asia, South America, and Africa, it is a popular folk medicine widely used for gastrointestinal ailments, influenza, nervous conditions, fever, coughs, pain, inflammation, and as a topical antiseptic.

> In tropical Asia, South America, and Africa, lemon grass is widely used for gastrointestinal ailments and numerous other conditions.

Current Use: Numerous scientific studies have been conducted on the chemistry and pharmacology of lemon grass. The essential oil has been found to have antifungal and antibacterial activity. One series of studies attempted to verify traditional uses such as the treatment of nervous and intestinal conditions, as well as fevers, but the researchers were unable to produce positive results with oral dosage forms. Diuretic and mild sedative effects have been confirmed in animal studies. Pharmacological data confirms carminative effects. Recent studies have shown lemon grass may have antimutagenic effects. Lemon grass is widely used as a folk medicine throughout Latin America to treat influenza, fevers, and stomachache.

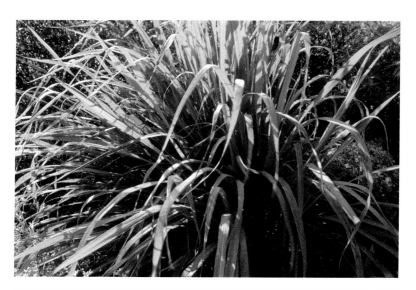

Used For:
Stomachache • Expelling gas

Preparations:
Dried leaf, cut and sifted.

Typical Dosage:
Tea: Steep 1 tsp dried herb in 1 cup hot water for 10–15 minutes. For commercial products, follow manufacturer's recommendations.

Cautions:
None noted.

Licorice

Glycyrrhiza glabra

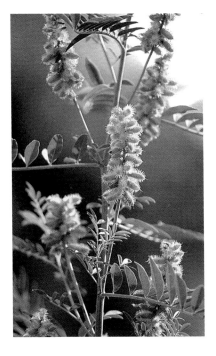

Sources: European licorice is the root of a member of the pea family native to, and commercially cultivated in Europe and Asia. Twenty species of *Glycyrrhiza* are found in Eurasia, North and South America, and Australia. At least six Chinese species, primarily *G. uralensis,* are used as Chinese licorice (*gan-cao* or sweet herb). Licorice is cultivated commercially in Europe and Asia.

Traditional Use: What we think of as "licorice" flavor is actually anise; licorice itself tastes very sweet and musty. The Roman naturalist Theophrastus (c. 372–287 B.C.) wrote that licorice roots were used for asthma, dry cough, and lung disorders. Traditionally, the dried root has also been used for sore throat and laryngitis as well as inflammation of the urinary and intestinal tracts. In China, it is used in prescriptions for coughs, sore throat, asthma, gastric and duodenal ulcers, and as a "mediator" of potentially toxic ingredients.

Current Use: Licorice is considered expectorant, diuretic, anti-inflammatory, and soothing to irritated mucous membranes; it is used in the treatment of inflamed lungs; it speeds healing of gastric and duodenal ulcers by increasing secretions from the gastric mucosa. Its cough-suppressant activity resembles that of codeine.

Glycyrrhizin (glycyrrhetic acid) is believed to be the primary active constituent, though other components of licorice contribute to its biological activity. Glycyrrhizin is fifty times as sweet as sugar and is found in licorice at concentrations of 1 to 25 percent. Good-quality licorice should contain at least 4 percent glycyrrhizin.

Licorice is one of the better-studied herbs. Numerous pharmacological and clinical reports confirm its usefulness in treating ulcers and support its reputation as a cough suppressant and expectorant. The German government allows licorice preparations to be used for the supportive treatment of gastric and duodenal ulcers and for congestion of the upper respiratory tract.

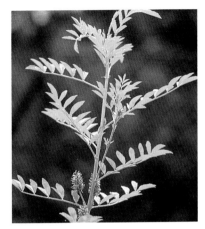

Used For:
Congestion • Coughs • Stomach or duodenal ulcers

Preparations:
Dried root whole, sliced, cut and sifted; capsules; extracts; tablets; tinctures; standardized products. European products are formulated to deliver 5–15 g (1–2 tsp) root, which contains 200–600 mg glycyrrhizin.

Typical Dosages:
Capsules: Up to six 400–500 mg capsules a day.
Tincture: 20–30 drops up to 3 times a day.
Or follow manufacturer's or practitioner's recommendations.

Cautions:
Licorice may cause some individuals to experience water retention and hypertension due to sodium retention and potassium loss. Do not exceed recommended dose. Discontinue use after four to six weeks. Individuals with heart disease, liver disease, or hypertension should avoid licorice, nor should licorice be used during pregnancy. If diuretics or heart medications containing digitalis have been prescribed, licorice should be avoided.

Marshmallow

Althaea officinalis

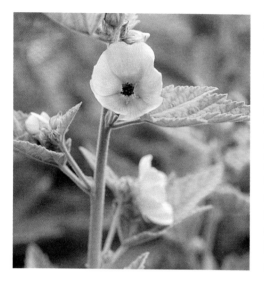

Sources: Marshmallow is the root or leaf of a member of the mallow family that grows in Europe from England, Denmark, and central Russia south to the Mediterranean region. Escaped from gardens in North America, it grows in salt marshes from Massachusetts to Virginia and in the mountains of the western United States. The root is used to a greater extent than the leaves.

Traditional Use: The genus name *Althaea* comes from the Greek *altho,* "associated with healing." Traditionally, marshmallow root has been poulticed on bruises, muscle aches, sprains, burns, and inflammations. A tea of the leaves has been used to soothe sore throat and upset stomach; as an expectorant it has been used for bronchitis and whooping cough. The leaves, both fresh and dried, are considered somewhat weaker.

> **Marshmallow preparations soothe and soften irritated tissue, particularly mucous membranes involved in sore throats accompanied by a dry cough.**

Current Use: The leaves and root both contain mucilagin, considered marshmallow's main active ingredient and the substance that makes the tea "slimy." The leaves contain up to 16 percent mucilagin, while the roots contain 25 to 30 percent. Marshmallow preparations are recognized for their ability to soothe and soften irritated tissue, particularly mucous membranes involved in sore throats accompanied by a dry cough. Marshmallow also mildly stimulates the immune system. The German health authorities allow use of leaf and root preparations for these purposes. Root preparations are also used to relieve local irritations, stimulate the immune system, slow down lung congestion in sore throat with dry cough, and relieve mild inflammation of the mucous membranes of the digestive tract.

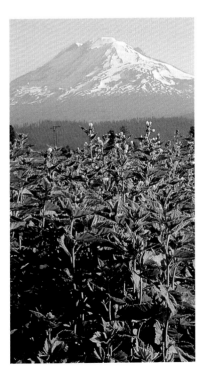

Used For:
Indigestion • Sore throats • Congestion • Expectorant

Preparations:
Whole or peeled root, cut and sifted or powdered; capsules, tablets, tinctures.

Typical Dosages:
Capsules: Up to six 400–500 mg capsules a day.
Tea: Steep 1–2 tsp dried leaves or 1 tsp dried root in 1 cup hot water for 10–15 minutes. Divide into 3 portions to use throughout the day.
Tincture: 20–40 drops up to 5 times a day.
Or follow manufacturer's or practitioner's recommendations.

Cautions:
The mucilagin in marshmallow may absorb and reduce the action of drugs taken at the same time. In Germany, the high sugar content of marshmallow syrups must be labeled to warn diabetics. No side effects are reported for marshmallow.

Milk Thistle

Silybum marianum

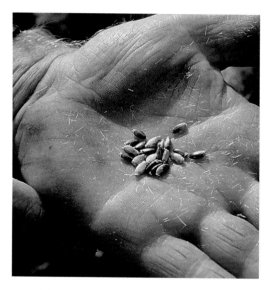

Source: Milk thistle is a member of the aster family found throughout Europe. Introduced by early colonists, it is naturalized in eastern North America and California. The seeds are used.

Traditional Use: According to early Greek references, milk thistle seeds have been used to treat liver disorders for more than 2,000 years. The Roman Pliny the Elder (A.D. 23–79), reported that the juice of the plant mixed with honey was excellent for "carrying off bile."

Milk thistle is featured in Hildegard of Bingen's *Physica,* the first herbal by a woman, written about 1150 and published in 1533; other early European herbals mention its use for liver disease. The sixteenth-century English herbalist John Gerard considered it "the best remedy that grows against all melancholy [liver] diseases," and the eighteenth-century German physician Rademacher used the seed for chronic and acute liver diseases. Its use declined over the next two centuries, but by the 1930s interest in using milk thistle for liver disease was growing again.

Current Use: More than 300 studies conducted since the late 1960s support the effectiveness and safety of silymarin, the main chemical complex in milk-thistle seeds, for treating liver disease. Standardized seed preparations have been shown to alter the cell structure of the outer liver membrane which prevents toxic chemicals from entering the liver and stimulates the liver's own capacity to generate new cells. Silymarin further protects the liver by scavenging harmful oxygen radicals.

German health authorities allow milk-thistle preparations to be used for chronic inflammatory liver disorders such as hepatitis, cirrhosis, and fatty infiltration caused by alcohol or other toxins. In addition to its well-documented curative actions, silymarin can help prevent liver damage when taken before exposure to toxins.

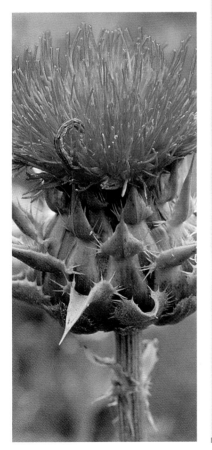

Used For:
Liver disorders

Preparations:
Whole or powdered seed, capsules, tablets, tinctures. Some products are standardized to 70–80% silymarin.

Typical Dosages:
Capsules: For standardized capsules, take 140 mg silymarin 3 times a day. After 6 weeks, reduce to 90 mg 3 times a day.
Tea: Steep 2–3 tsp dried, powdered seed in 1 cup hot water for 10–15 minutes.
Tincture: 10–25 drops up to 3 times a day.
Or follow manufacturer's or practitioner's recommendations.

Cautions:
No serious side effects, contraindications, or drug interactions have been reported for milk-thistle preparations. Loose stools may occur during the first few days of use.

Motherwort

Leonurus cardiaca

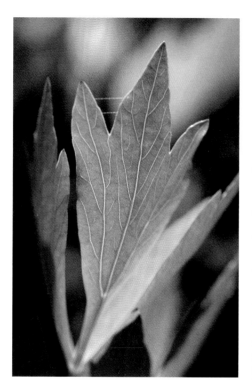

Sources: European motherwort, *Leonurus cardiaca,* found throughout much of Europe, has become naturalized in the United States and is a common weed in many parts of the country. The northeast Asian species, *L. sibericus,* is also naturalized (though much less frequently) in the Pacific Northwest, Texas, and the Gulf Coast. It and other Asian species are the source of an ancient Chinese herb, *yi-mu-cao (i-mu-ts'ao [L. artemisia]).* For the American market, motherwort harvested in flower is imported from Europe. Chinese preparations employ both herb and seeds.

Traditional Use: Whenever different cultures on opposite sides of the world use closely-related plants for similar or identical purposes, strong probability of a rational scientific lies behind that use. In both Europe and China, motherwort is used to promote blood circulation and regulate the menses, and as a diuretic. In Europe, motherwort is also employed as a mild sedative and astringent, and is valued for relieving spasms and lowering blood pressure. In China, motherwort is used to reduce swelling and stimulate development of new tissue.

Current Use: In a country where heart disease is still the number-one killer, it is amazing that the historical use of both European and Asian motherworts in the management of heart disease has sparked little interest or research. Chinese researchers have found that the herb or its extracts increase the volume of blood circulation, stimulate uterine activity, and promote urine flow. Clinical reports from China (though not controlled clinical studies in the modern sense) have confirmed positive results in use of the herb to treat heart disease, hypertension, irregular menstruation, excessive menstrual bleeding, and kidney disease. In the West, motherwort is considered sedative, hypotensive, and cardiotonic. Recent preliminary research indicates the possibility of antioxidant, immunostimulating, and cancer preventive activity.

Used For:
Cardiac symptoms associated with nervous conditions • Menstrual difficulties • Spasms

Preparations:
Dried herb, cut and sifted or powdered; tincture.

Typical Dosages:
Tea: Steep 1/2 to 1 tsp in 1 cup hot water for 10–15 minutes. Use 3 times a day.
Tincture: 20–50 drops up to 5 times a day.
Or follow manufacturer's or practitioner's recommendations.

Cautions:
Since motherwort is known as a cardiotonic, it should be used only under a physician's supervision if other cardiac drugs are prescribed. Avoid use during pregnancy and nursing. It is known that the herb affects the uterus; however, there are no toxicity studies. The few reports of toxic reactions in the literature relate to rare contact dermatitis from handling the plant.

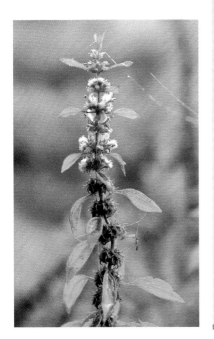

Mullein

Verbascum thapsus

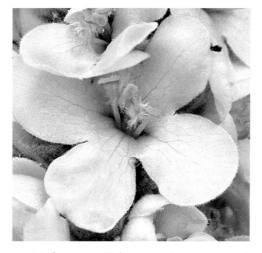

Sources: Mullein, a member of the figwort family, has great claim to fame as a weed. Native to Eurasia, it is found throughout much of Europe and Asia and is naturalized throughout North America. Both the leaves and flowers are used medicinally. The herb is commercially harvested in both Europe and the United States. There are over 360 species of *Verbascum*. Other species commonly used in herbal traditions include *V. phlomoides* and *V. densiflorum* (*V. thapsiforme*), which also occur in North America.

Traditional Use: Historically, mullein is primarily used for lung conditions and as an expectorant. The dried leaves have been smoked like tobacco to relieve lung congestion and irritation of the mucous membranes. Mullein cigarettes have been especially valued for treatment of asthma and spasmodic coughs, though asthmatics are best advised not to smoke anything. Traditionally, the flowers, soaked in olive oil, have served as a folk treatment for earache and inflammatory conditions of the mucous membranes. Externally, both the leaves and flowers have been used for treating wounds. In India, mullein is used as a folk medicine for inflammatory disease, asthma, spasmodic coughs, and migraine.

Current Use: Despite scant scientific evidence of efficacy, mullein leaves and flowers continue to enjoy use for their traditional applications, particularly the leaves for lung conditions and a macerated oil of the flowers for earache. Mucilage has been found in both the flowers and the leaves, along with various iridoids, saponins, and flavonoids, all of which could contribute to biological activity.

Antiviral activity has been reported in laboratory studies against influenza and *Herpes simplex* viruses, along with mild expectorant activity. Mullein flowers are preferred over the leaves in European phytomedicine. The German regulatory authorities allow use of mullein flowers as a soothing expectorant in catarrh of the upper respiratory tract. Both flowers and leaves are used in numerous cough and bronchial phytomedicines in Europe.

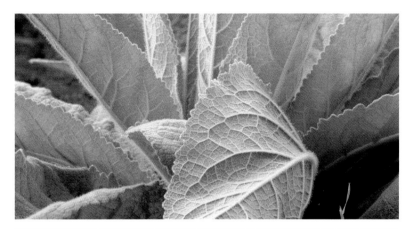

Used For:
Catarrhs of the upper respiratory tract • Earache

Preparations:
Dried flowers and leaves, whole or cut and sifted; capsules, tablets, tinctures, flowers in olive oil.

Typical Dosages:
Tea: Steep 2 tsp dried flowers and leaves in 1 cup hot water for 10–15 minutes. Use up to 6–8 times a day.
Tincture: 25–40 drops every 3 hours.
Or follow manufacturer's or practitioner's recommendations.

Cautions:
None noted.

Neem

Azadirachta indica

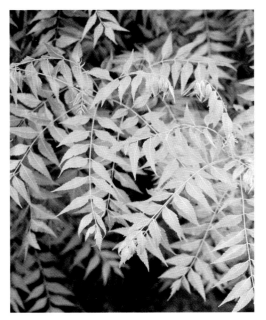

Sources: A tree of the mahogany family known as "free tree," perhaps for its ability to unleash nutrients from arid subsoil on poor arid lands, hence "freeing" the soil, neem occurs throughout much of southern and southeast Asia. It is widely cultivated in arid areas of Africa, the Middle East, and Central and South America. It is also grown in Hawaii and southern Florida. All parts of the plant are used.

Traditional Use: Virtually all parts of the plant have been used in folk and traditional medicine in India, and these uses have filled several books. The young tender branches have been used as chewing sticks (toothbrushes); the leaf's essential oil has been used as a local antiseptic and insecticide; a poultice of the leaves has been used for swollen glands, bruises, and sprains. In tropical regions, the bitter fresh-leaf tea has been used as a folk medicine for malaria. Both tree and root barks have been used in India since ancient times for the treatment of malaria, jaundice, and to expel worms. The pulp of the fruit is considered edible and is used medicinally for urinary diseases and to treat hemorrhoids. The seeds, perhaps the most useful part of the tree, produce a bitter fixed oil known as "Oil of Margosa" or neem oil.

Current Use: Dr. Paul Hoversten of the National Research Council hailed the virtues of neem in a 1995 article in *USA Today.* Neem, he states, "may eventually benefit every person on the planet. The plant may usher in a new era in pest control, provide millions with inexpensive medicine, cut down the rate of human population growth and perhaps even reduce erosion, deforestation, and the excessive temperature of an overheated globe."

Neem is a veritable chemical factory. Neem extracts are used in commercial toothpastes. Limited trials have shown that neem oil is potentially useful against gingivitis. Leaf extracts have been shown to have antiviral activity and delay blood clotting (useful for snakebite); the leaves' essential oil has been shown to have strong antibacterial and antifungal activity. Both antifungal and antiseptic, the seed oil has been used as an ingredient in dentifrices) and is being researched for antifertility potential. The fresh seed oil has a strong garlic-like odor and is used as an ingredient in insect sprays. Neem-leaf products are used similarly to goldenseal, as a mild antibacterial and antiviral natural product.

Used For:
Gingivitis • Mild mouth infections • Fighting bacteria, fungi, and viruses • Repelling insects

Preparations:
Dried leaf, cut and sifted or powdered; neem seed oil, capsules.

Typical Dosage:
Capsules: Up to six 400–500 mg capsules a day.
Or follow manufacturer's or practitioner's recommendations.

Cautions:
Seed oil and seed extracts in insecticides are considered safe for mammals in concentrations approved for use. Neem oil (either seed oil or essential oil) should not be ingested. Leaf products should be used only on a short-term basis. There are unconfirmed reports that long-term use for malaria in Africa has led to kidney failure. Use all neem products only as directed.

Nopal

Opuntia ficus-indica and other *Opuntia* spp.

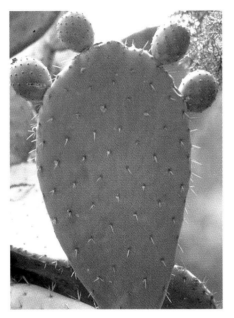

Sources: *Opuntia,* also known as prickly pear, is a large genus in the cactus family with over 300 species. *Opuntia ficus-indica,* native to Mexico, was taken to Europe at an early date and is now common in many warmer regions of the world, including North Africa, Mediterranean Europe, India, South and Central America, and the western United States. Commercial supplies come from Mexico and elsewhere. Nopal is the ancient Aztec name for prickly pear.

Traditional Use: When Spaniards first arrived in Mexico, the Aztecs were already cultivating nopal in orchards for the edible fruits. The first reference to nopal comes from the oldest medical book from the Americas, *The Badianus Manuscript,* or Aztec Herbal of 1552. The word *Nohpalli,* or nopal, is derived from the Latinization of the Aztec name *tlatocnochtli.* The milky juice from the cactus, mixed with other herbs, was combined with honey and egg yolk as an ointment to treat burns.

Subsequently introduced to India by Portuguese traders three centuries ago, nopal fruits are used as food and to make a syrup for whooping cough and asthma.

In China, the fresh pad of the cactus has been used as a dressing on abscesses. Cooked alone or with pork, its broth strengthens weak patients; fried with eggs, it treats numbness. The pads were dried under the sun, pounded into coarse pieces, and mixed with oil for curing a scalded head. In Italy and North Africa, nopal flowers are used as a strong diuretic. In Mexican folk medicine, the pads are used for diabetes, high cholesterol, and obesity. The flowers have also been used for treating benign prostatic hyperplasia.

Current Use: Recent scientific interest in nopal stems from Mexican studies published in the late 1980s. The researchers found that after fasting for twelve hours, patients with noninsulin dependent diabetes who were given nopal had lower blood-glucose and higher insulin levels. Researchers theorized that the cactus leaves may improve the effectiveness of available insulin. More research will have to be conducted to assess nopal's potential value in treating noninsulin dependent diabetes.

A recent Israeli study examined the potential of preparations of dried flowers in treating benign prostatic hyperplasia. This preliminary trial reported significant reduction in the urge to urinate. The encouraging results have prompted a larger controlled study in progress.

Used For:
Diuresis • Benign prostatic hypertrophy • Folk medicine for diabetes

Preparations:
Dried pads, flowers; fruits; capsules, dried extracts, tablets.

Typical Dosages:
Dried extract: 250 mg 2 times a day.
Fresh leaf pad: 1 oz a day.
(No therapeutic dosage has been established. The above quantities were used in clinical studies in Mexico. For commercial products, follow manufacturer's recommendations.)

Cautions:
Diabetics seeking alternative therapies should consult their health-care practitioner before using nopal.

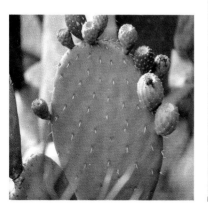

Oatstraw

Avena sativa

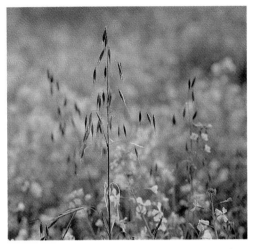

Sources: Oatstraw comes from the same plant as the rolled oats in your breakfast oatmeal. Native to the Mediterranean region, oats were cultivated in much of Europe by 2000 B.C. The straw left from harvest of the grains is the herbal oatstraw of commerce.

Traditional Use: Oatmeal has been traditionally considered a nutritive and demulcent, once prescribed for habitual constipation. As gruel, it was served to convalescing patients. Oatstraw arose as an important nerve tonic and antispasmodic in nineteenth-century medicines used for spasm and nervous disorders accompanied by exhaustion and other forms of nervous debility. It was considered useful for spasmodic conditions of the bladder and debility produced by chronic conditions. Used in baths, oats are a folk remedy for arthritis, rheumatism, and skin disorders. In the nineteenth century, an oats patent medicine was promoted as a treatment for morphine addiction. In modern herbalism, that has translated into a treatment for tobacco addiction.

> **Oatstraw is approved in Germany for application to inflammatory skin conditions involving itching.**

Current Use: In European phytotherapy, oatstraw, primarily in the form of a tincture or tea from the green tops, is valued as a diuretic. It is also said to lower uric acid levels in the blood. No scientific research confirms traditional use as an antispasmodic and nervine, nor have active constituents been identified. Despite the apparent lack of pharmacological and clinical research, oatstraw is approved by the German health authorities for application to inflammatory skin eruptions involving itching. It is usually used in a bath.

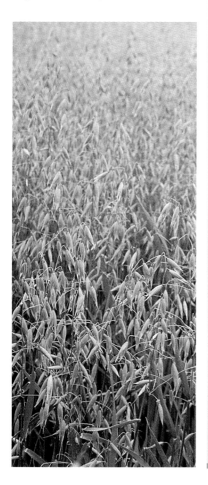

Used For:
Diuresis • Reducing inflammation and itching

Preparations:
Dried herb; capsules, tablets, tinctures.

Typical Dosages:
Bath: 4 oz dried tops in a tub of hot water.

Tea: Steep 1 tbsp dried tops in 1 cup hot water for 10–15 minutes.

For commercial products, follow manufacturer's recommendations.

Tincture: 25 drops 3 times a day.

Or follow manufacturer's or practitioner's recommendations.

Cautions:
None noted.

Olive Leaf

Olea europea

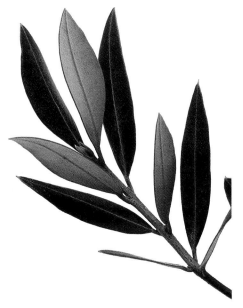

Sources: In recent years, interest has been sparked in using olive leaf as a dietary supplement. Given the fact that olives have been grown in the Mediterranean since the dawn of history, it is no wonder that olive growers, at some early date, also tried a tea of the leaves.

Traditional Use: Traditionally, olive leaf has been valued as an astringent and antiseptic. A decoction of the leaves is made by boiling two handsful of the leaves in a quart of water, then simmering to half the original volume. This brew is used to treat fevers. The tea is also used as a mild diuretic and to treat malaria. Externally, the leaves are poulticed to treat boils, skin rashes, and sprains.

Current Use: Scientists first isolated a compound called oleuropein from olive leaf in the late 1800s. This compound has strong antibacterial and antifungal activity and occurs throughout the tree, usually at levels of up to 0.3 percent in the leaf. The compound is believed to help protect the tree from insect attack and disease and olive oil from spoilage. A number of European studies have found that the leaf extracts have strong antioxidant activity and may benefit the nervous system and help protect against aging and cardiovascular disease. Since olives themselves have higher levels of oleuropein, olive-leaf extract may be attractive to individuals who don't like olives. No olive product is allowed to carry therapeutic claims in Germany for lack of scientific evidence.

Used For:
General well-being

Preparations:
Dried leaf; extracts containing 6–15% oleuropein.

Typical Dosage:
Tea: Steep 1 tsp dried leaves in 1 cup hot water for 10–15 minutes. (Dosage is not well-established. For commercial products, follow manufacturer's recommendations.)

Cautions:
Olive leaf has been reported to irritate the digestive tract if taken on an empty stomach. Both fruit and leaves can cause rare cases of skin rashes.

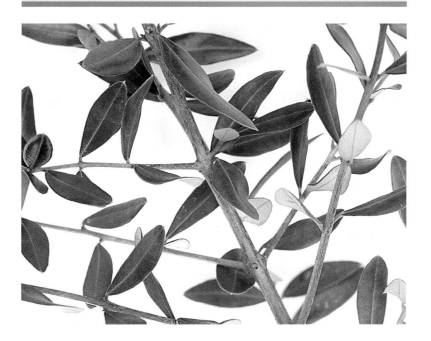

Parsley

Petroselinum crispum

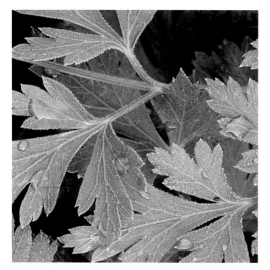

Sources: Best known as the curled green sprig decorating your plate at restaurants and usually still on the plate when you're done, parsley is a member of the carrot family native to Europe. Some varieties produce wavy or curled leaves; Italian parsley is flat-leaved. In Europe, certain varieties are grown for their roots. At one time or another, the leaves, seeds, and the roots have all been used as herbal remedies. The leaves are collected in the second year of growth before flowering.

Traditional Use: Use of parsley is not limited to plates. The leaves, both fresh and dried, have a reputation as a breath freshener and are valued as a diuretic. Parsley root was used by nineteenth-century practitioners for dropsy (water retention) and gonorrhea. The bruised fresh leaves were used as a poultice for contusions, enlarged glands, and insect bites. The dried powdered leaves were sprinkled on the hair or used in the form of an ointment to kill head lice. The roots were also considered diuretic. Traditionally, parsley leaf tea has been used to soothe painful menstruation.

Current Use: In European phytomedicine, parsley leaves are used as a carminative to relieve flatulence and as a diuretic. In Germany, parsley-leaf preparations are approved for treating lower urinary tract infections and gravel in the kidneys. Parsley seed is not approved for use in Germany because its traditional uses have not been substantiated and because it has demonstrated relatively high risk factors. In France, parsley leaf is used in topical preparations for soothing itchy, cracked, or chapped skin. It is also allowed for use in painful menstrual periods. One component of parsley leaf oil, myristicin, is being researched for possible cancer-preventing activity.

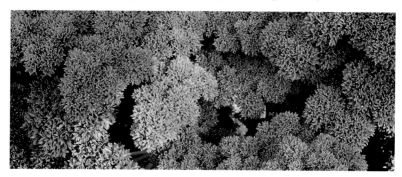

Used For:
Diuresis • Painful menstruation

Preparations:
Fresh, dried, or freeze-dried leaf; capsules, tincture.

Typical Dosages:
Capsules: Up to six 400–500 mg capsules a day.
Fresh herb: Eat at will.
Tea: Steep 2 tsp dried herb in 1 cup hot water for 10–15 minutes. Use up to 3 times a day.
Tincture: 30–60 drops up to 3 times a day.
Or follow manufacturer's or practitioner's recommendations.

Cautions:
According to German health authorities, parsley leaf is contraindicated during pregnancy and inflammation of the kidneys. Contact dermatitis, allergic skin reactions, or reactions with the mucous membranes are possible, though rare. Light-skinned individuals may experience photodermatitis. In pregnant women, use of parsley seed is not recommended because the contractions it causes can lead to abortion. The seeds can also cause bleeding and inflammation of the mucosal linings of the gastrointestinal tract.

Peppermint

Mentha ✕piperita

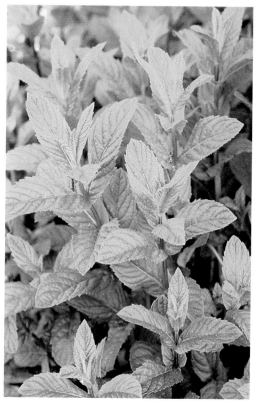

Source: Peppermint is the leaf of a hybrid between spearmint (*Mentha spicata*) and watermint (*M. aquatica*). Native to Europe, it was first grown commercially in England about 1750. Today peppermint is produced commercially in Indiana, Wisconsin, Oregon, Washington, and Idaho.

Traditional Use: Peppermint is first mentioned in the medical literature of the early 1700s. Samuel Stern described it in 1801 in *The American Herbal:* "It is a stimulant. It restores the functions of the stomach, promotes digestion, stops vomiting, cures the hiccups, flatulent colic, hysterical depressions, and other like complaints." Peppermint leaf tea has been used traditionally for indigestion, nausea, colds, headache, and cramps.

Current Use: Recent research on peppermint has concentrated on its essential oil, 30 to 48 percent of which is menthol. Peppermint oil has been shown to be antibacterial and antiviral; it also reduces muscle spasms.

Recent research shows that peppermint oil is effective in treating irritable bowel syndrome only when administered in coated capsules that permit the oil to reach the colon without first being digested in the stomach. Inhalation of peppermint essential oil is thought to ease congestion from colds and improve breathing by stimulating cold receptors in the respiratory tract. In its 1990 review of over-the-counter drugs, the FDA dropped peppermint oil from its former status as a nonprescription drug, most likely because no data on its safety or effectiveness had been submitted by the industry. Peppermint oil is still widely used and approved in Europe.

Used For:
Gastrointestinal spasms • Nausea • Congestion

Preparations:
Dried leaf, cut and sifted; enteric coated capsules of peppermint oil, tinctures.

Typical Dosages:
Oil: 6–12 drops in water 3 times a day. For respiratory congestion, put a few drops in a basin of hot water and inhale the vapor with your eyes closed.
Oil capsules: 1 to 2 capsules 3 times a day between meals.
Tea: Steep 2–4 tsp dried, cut and sifted leaf in 1½–3 cups hot water for 15 minutes. Take throughout the day as needed.
Tincture: 10–20 drops in water after meals.
Or follow manufacturer's or practitioner's recommendations. Do not exceed recommended dosages.

Cautions:
Coated peppermint-oil capsules may sometimes open in the stomach, causing heartburn and relaxation of throat muscles. They should not be used by anyone diagnosed with an absence of hydrochloric acid in their gastric juices (achlorhydria). Peppermint oil should not be applied directly to the mucous membranes, especially the nostrils of infants and children. The leaf and oil should not be used by anyone with gallbladder or bile-duct obstruction, inflammation, or related conditions.

Plantain

Plantago major and *P. lanceolata*

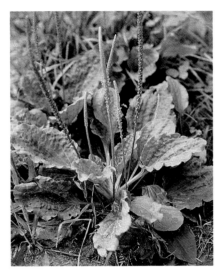

Sources: The plantain family contains upwards of 270 species, many more commonly classified as "weeds" than herbs. Common plantain, *Plantago major*, and English or lance-leaved plantain, *P. lanceolata*, are native to Eurasia but widely naturalized. They occur throughout North America and are common on lawns. Wherever plants grow, one can find plantain. Psyllium seed comes from other *Plantago* species (see Psyllium seed).

Traditional Use: Bruised or crushed plantain leaves are a common folk remedy for bites, insect stings, ulcers, eczema, and many other skin ailments. They have also been used to stop localized bleeding of small wounds or cuts. In the form of tea the leaves are historically considered diuretic, anti-inflammatory, antiseptic, and cooling. They have been used for menstrual difficulties, diarrhea, dysentery, hemorrhoids, and lung ailments, and to help break up phlegm in the upper respiratory tract. Plantain leaves are used in folk medicine wherever they grow, from Europe to Asia to South and North America.

Current Use: Much chemical work has been done on these two species of plantain, identifying numerous compounds that may be involved in biological activity. Animal experiments have shown that a water extract of the leaves has a toning effect on uterine muscles. One compound may be responsible for documented liver-protective effects. Several Eastern European clinical studies have confirmed use in chronic bronchitis, while another suggests effectiveness in treating bronchial symptoms associated with colds. Plantain has also been shown to have wound-healing and mild antibiotic and anti-inflammatory activity.

In Germany, *P. lanceolata* is allowed for its soothing, astringent, and antibacterial action in catarrhs of the upper respiratory tract and inflamed mucous membranes of the mouth and throat. Externally, it is used on skin inflammations. Potential cancer-preventing activity has also been suggested. Plantain is certainly an herb for which further research is justified.

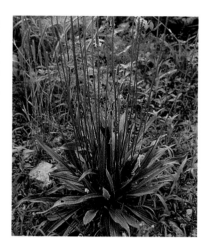

Used For:
Bronchitis • Catarrhs of the upper respiratory tract • Insect bites or stings

Preparations:
Dried herb; capsules, tablets. Used in multiherb formulas.

Typical Dosage:
Tea: Steep 2 tsp dried herb in 1 cup hot water for 10–15 minutes. Repeat 3 to 4 times a day as needed.
Or follow manufacturer's or practitioner's recommendations.

Cautions:
No side effects, contraindications, or drug interactions are generally listed for plantain. In rare instances, contact dermatitis may occur in sensitive individuals. Cross reactivity with psyllium has been documented; people using plantain should avoid bulk laxatives containing psyllium seed. Reports of toxicity linked to imported "plantain leaves" has resulted from misidentification of or contamination with the leaves of *Digitalis lanata,* a source of the heart stimulator digitalis. These reports have resulted in closer attention to botanical and chemical identification of the raw materials.

Prickly Ash

Zanthoxylum americanum and *Z. clava-herculis*

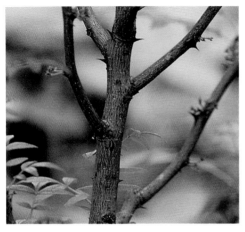

Sources: Prickly ash is the bark of either the northern prickly ash (*Zanthoxylum americanum*) or southern prickly ash (*Z. clava-herculis*), members of the rue family. Over 250 species in the genus are found in the Americas, Africa, and Australia. Several Asian species are used in the traditional medicine of China and Japan. Northern prickly ash is a tall shrub found in moist woods from Quebec to Georgia, west to Oklahoma, and north to Ohio. Southern prickly ash, also known as Hercules' club, is found in damp woods from Delaware south to Florida and west to Texas and Arkansas. Southern prickly ash is most abundant in Texas, the source of most of the commercial supply.

Traditional Use: Early American physicians considered the properties of the two species of prickly ash to be identical, and the bark was one of the most widely used herbs in nineteenth-century medicine. Native Americans used it to treat toothaches, hence the name "toothache tree." The eminent American naturalist, Thomas Nuttall, notes the use of prickly ash for toothaches in his travels through the Arkansas territory in 1819. Chewing the bark enhanced the flow of saliva and gastric and intestinal juice output; therefore, the herb was deemed valuable for stimulating digestion, bile secretions, and pancreatic activity. Bark was widely used for rheumatic conditions and for nervous conditions accompanied by mouth dryness to "stimulate" the mucous membranes. A tea of the bark was used for uterine cramps, neuralgia, fevers, and enhancing circulation.

Current Use: Very little scientific research has been conducted on the two North American species of prickly ash. Most research in the literature relates to Asian and African species, with anti-inflammatory, antibacterial, and cardiovascular benefits identified. Research on isolated components in the bark of southern prickly ash shows antibacterial and anti-inflammatory activity. One study found that extracts of the bark of southern prickly ash affect muscle contractility by blocking or stimulating neuromuscular transmissions. These studies were prompted by observation of toxic effects in cattle that had grazed on the branches. Prickly ash contains a number of alkaloids and alkalmides, one of which, neo-herculin, produces a local numbing effect. It is believed to be identical in structure to echinacein, a component in echinacea responsible for the numbing sensation the roots produce on the tongue. Prickly ash preparations are used in European phytomedicines for treating rheumatic conditions and Raynaud's disease, and to stimulate circulation for intermittent claudication. Prickly ash is in serious need of more research.

Used For:
Bronchitis • Rheumatism • Healing

Preparations:
Bark, whole, cut and sifted, powdered; capsules, tablets, tinctures.

Typical Dosages:
Tea: Steep 1 tsp bark in a cup of hot water for 10–15 minutes. Take up to 3 times a day.
Tincture (bark): 10–30 drops.
Tincture (berries): 5–15 drops before meals.
Or follow manufacturer's or practitioner's recommendations.

Cautions:
Given its traditional use as a uterine stimulant, prickly ash should be avoided during pregnancy. More research is needed.

Psyllium

Plantago spp.

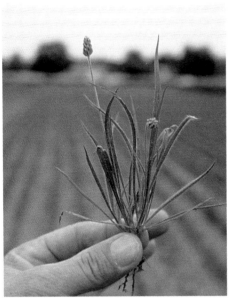

Sources: Psyllium seeds and husks come from two annual species of plantain, a plant group familiar to most as lawn weeds. Blonde psyllium, native to the Mediterranean, North Africa, and western Asia, is widely grown in India and Pakistan. Black psyllium (*Plantago psyllium* and *P. indica,* both known as *P. arenaria*) is also native to the Mediterranean region and is commercially grown in Spain and southern France.

Traditional Use: The seeds and husks of psyllium have long been used as bulk laxatives in Europe and the United States.

Current Use: Many consumers may already have psyllium-seed products on their shelves because psyllium is a common ingredient in bulk laxatives. The seeds and seed husks contain 10 to 30 percent mucilage and, when soaked in water, increase greatly in volume to swell the amount of intestinal matter. This action stimulates and lubricates the bowels, encouraging the movement of wastes through the colon. Psyllium-seed products are widely prescribed and are also available as nonprescription drugs

> **Many consumers may already have psyllium-seed products on their shelf because psyllium is a common ingredient in bulk laxatives.**

for the treatment of chronic constipation or to soften the stool to relieve hemorrhoids and related conditions.

In Germany the seeds and husks are allowed in the supportive treatment of irritable bowel syndrome. Studies have shown that psyllium produces a modest but significant reduction in cholesterol levels.

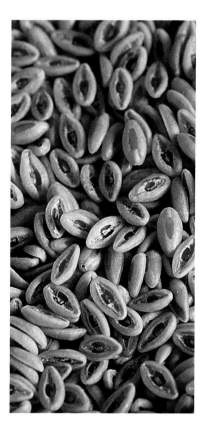

Used For:
Constipation • Lowering cholesterol

Preparations:
Dried seed, husk; capsules.

Typical Dosages:
Capsules: Take up to six 660 mg capsules a day. Take a full glass of water with each dose.
Whole herb: Stir up to 1 tsp of husks or 2 tsp powdered seed in a large glass of water and drink immediately 30 minutes to an hour after meals or after taking other drugs.
Or follow manufacturer's or practitioner's recommendations.

Cautions:
According to German health authorities, psyllium seeds and husks are known to produce rare allergic reactions and can be dangerous in cases of intestinal obstruction. Because some psyllium preparations contain sugar, diabetics should use them only under a physician's supervision.

Pygeum

Prunus africana (Syn. *Pygeum africanum*)

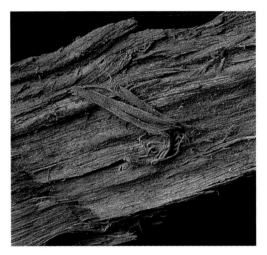

Sources: Pygeum is the bark of an African tree (a member of the rose family) that grows in highland mountain forest "islands" and is harvested commercially in the center of the continent and on Madagascar as well as the Democratic Republic of Congo, Kenya, and Zaire. Much of pygeum's habitat has been lost to clear-cutting. Over-exploitation has resulted in conservation concerns and the species being listed in Appendix II of the Convention on International Trade in Endangered Species (CITES) in order to monitor the impact of international trade.

Traditional Use: In African counties, pygeum bark is used by traditional healers for inflammation, kidney disease, malaria, stomachache, and fever. Closely related to cherries (also a member of the rose family), the fruits are small and very bitter. The freshly cut bark, fresh crushed leaves, and fruits all contain hydrocyanic acid, which has a strong cherry or almond fragrance. In Natal the bark was traditionally made into milk tea to treat difficult urination.

Current Use: Like the fruit of saw palmetto and the root of stinging nettle, the bark of pygeum is valued in European phytotherapy for the treatment of benign prostatic hypertrophy (BPH), a nonmalignant enlargement of the prostate which afflicts most men over fifty years old. Three classes of chemical constituents have been found in non-water extracts: phytosterols, triterpenes, and organic acids which produce a beneficial effect on the prostate. This includes anti-inflammatory activity, a reduction of cholesterol levels in the prostate, and inhibition of prostaglandin synthesis. In 1966, a patent was issued for use of the bark extract in the treatment of benign prostatic hypertrophy. Over the past two decades, twenty-six clinical trials on pygeum extracts, at a dose of 100 to 200 mg a day, have shown positive effects in the treatment of BPH symptoms such as difficult urination, frequent nighttime urination, and volume of residual urine. Pharmacological studies have shown that pygeum may increase prostate secretions, thus improving the composition of seminal fluid and perhaps sexual function. Most research and clinical experiments have been done in Italy and France, rather than Germany. Pygeum is often used in combination with stinging nettle root and/or saw palmetto extracts. Its future will depend upon development of sustainable supply.

Used For:
Reducing inflammation • Benign prostatic hypertrophy (BPH)

Preparations:
Bark, whole, cut and sifted, powdered; capsules, tablets, tinctures. Standardized to 14% triterpenes and 0.5% n-docosanol.

Typical Dosage:
For standardized products, the dose is 100–200 mg a day. Or follow manufacturer's or practitioner's recommendations.

Cautions:
Gastrointestinal irritation, including nausea and stomach pain, has been reported in clinical trials. Since BPH is not self-limiting or self-diagnosable, it should be treated under a physician's supervision.

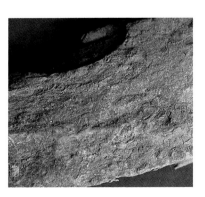

Raspberry Leaves

Rubus idaeus

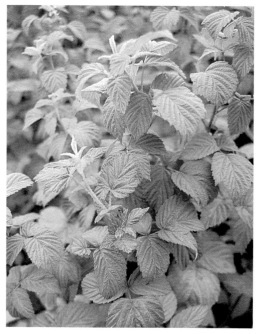

Sources: Raspberry fruits are famous, but the leaves are also valued in herbal medicine. *Rubus idaeus,* the common raspberry, is a highly variable plant group found in Eurasia and North America. Most of the supply comes from Europe.

Traditional Use: The astringent properties of raspberry leaf tea have been valued for the treatment of diarrhea, stomach ailments, tonsillitis, conjunctivitis, dysentery, menstrual cramps, fevers, colds, and flu. The tea has also been used for more than two millennia to treat wounds. The primary use in modern herbal traditions is to facilitate childbirth, with the tea drunk throughout pregnancy to treat morning sickness, reduce risk of miscarriage. and lessen labor pains by strengthening the uterus.

Current Use: Little research has been conducted on raspberry leaves, yet the tea is prescribed for pregnant women by many lay and professional midwives. Rudimentary work has been done on the chemistry, showing the leaves contain flavonoids, tannins, and various organic acids, constituents ubiquitous to many plants. Several interesting pharmacological studies suggest more research should be conducted. An extract of the leaves has been reported to have little effect on uterine muscles of laboratory animals, yet in pregnant rats it inhibited contraction of uterine muscles. One report states that it produces more regular, less frequent contractions. A compound has been identified that stimulates smooth-muscle action, especially of the uterine muscle. Another fraction was found that reduced uterine contractions. With no controlled studies to support these traditional uses, therapeutic claims are not allowed in Germany. Nevertheless, there is probably no herb in the American market that has been used by as many pregnant women as raspberry leaf tea. Unidentified hormonal activity could be responsible. Certainly this is a plant in need of research.

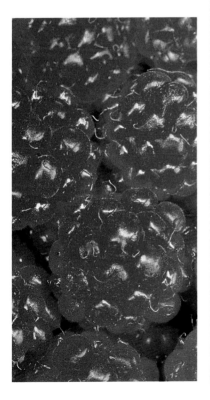

Used For:
Astringent • A folk tonic during pregnancy • Diarrhea

Preparations:
Dried leaf, cut and sifted or powdered; capsules, tablets, tinctures. (Tinctures may contain other components.)

Typical Dosages:
Capsules: Up to six 430 mg capsules a day.
Tea: Steep 1 tsp dried leaves in 1 cup hot water for 10 to 15 minutes. Use as often as 10 times a day.
Or follow manufacturer's or practitioner's recommendations.

Cautions:
Laboratory experiments show that raspberry leaf tea affects the uterus. Because the exact nature of the effect is unknown, the tea should be used during pregnancy only under experienced medical supervision.

Red Clover

Trifolium pratense

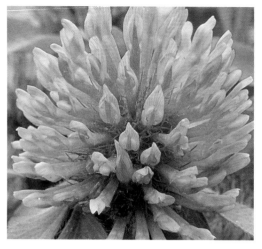

Source: Red clover is the dried flower head of a member of the pea family widely grown as animal fodder in temperate climates of the world. It is native to Europe and naturalized throughout the United States.

Traditional Use: Red clover is mentioned as a blood purifier, diuretic, general tonic, and folk cancer remedy in Jethro Kloss's *Back to Eden*. The flower has been used as a folk remedy to relieve spasms associated with asthma and bronchitis and to treat sores or ulcerations. It is one of the ingredients of the controversial Hoxsy, a formula used at alternative cancer clinics in Mexico.

Current Use: Red clover's use as a cancer remedy is not backed by any clinical studies in humans. The herb does, however, contain isoflavones that have estrogenic activity, including genistein, diadzen, formononetin, and biochanin A. Those that bind with estrogen receptors in the body are known as phenolic phytoestrogens (phyto means plant; estrogen is a naturally occurring hormone). Phytoestrogens activate estrogen receptors in mammals. Increasingly phytoestrogenic isoflavones are recognized as significant natural sources of complementary estrogens for humans. Red clover is the richest source of these compounds. Phytoestrogen isoflavonoids have attracted the attention of epidemiologists who believe that semivegetarian diets of Asian countries help account for their much lower incidence of breast, colorectal, and prostate cancer.

Epidemiological studies provide evidence that certain dietary components can have a significant effect on the incidence and location of cancers in humans, and James A. Duke is one herbal-health professional who suggests that red clover is a good candidate for further study as a dietary substance that may help prevent cancer. It is already known that some members of the mustard family, especially broccoli, help prevent the development of cancers, an effect attributed to their ability to scavenge free radicals. The flavonoid genistein (mostly extracted from soybeans) is now available in dietary supplements. A recent preliminary laboratory study found that biochanin A inhibited the activation of cancer in cell cultures. More research on red clover and its isoflavones is clearly warranted.

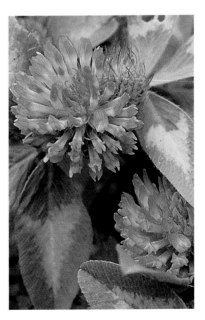

Used For:
Cancer prevention • Estrogen source

Preparations:
Dried tops.

Typical Dosages:
Capsules: Up to five 430 mg capsules a day.
Tea: Steep 1 tbsp in a cup of hot water for 10–15 minutes.
Tincture: 15–30 drops up to 4 times a day.
Or follow manufacturer's or practitioner's recommendations.

Cautions:
No side effects have been reported from using this herb. However, cattle ingesting late-season or spoiled red clover hay have developed symptoms such as frothing, diarrhea, dermatitis, and decreased milk production. It is possible that similar effects could occur in persons using fermented or otherwise spoiled red clover.

Reishi

Ganoderma lucidum

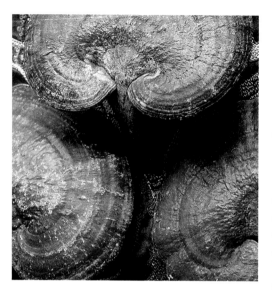

Sources: Known as *reishi* in Japan or *ling-zhi* in China, this herb is the fruiting body of a mushroom. It is produced commercially in China, Japan, and the United States. In Japan it grows in the wild on plum trees, but most of the supply is cultivated. Related species such as artist's conk (*Ganoderma applanatum*) occur in North America, but they are not grown commercially nor have their medicinal properties been studied.

Traditional Use: Reishi has been a folk medicine in China for thousands of years. It is mentioned in the first class of herbs in *Shen Nong Ben Cao Jing* for calming, benefiting vital energy (Qi), and even improving the complexion. Once available only to emperors, this important tonic was considered an "elixir of life" and was used in Traditional Chinese Medicine (TCM) to treat hepatitis, hypertension, arthritis, nervous conditions, insomnia, lung disorders, and as a general tonic to "lighten weight and increase longevity."

Current Use: Reishi's activity is ascribed not to one chemical, but to the collective action of many components, including polysaccharides, whose immunostimulant activity helps enhance protein synthesis; a heart-toning alkaloid; and triterpene acids which protect the liver, reduce hypertension, and inhibit cholesterol synthesis. Pharmacological studies have confirmed that reishi is anti-allergenic, anti-inflammatory, antiviral, antioxidant, immunostimulant, and expectorant, and that it suppresses coughs and increases coronary blood flow. In the past two decades, Asian clinical studies have shown that reishi is effective in treating hepatitis, lowering cholesterol, and relieving bronchitis and asthma. It is also effective in relieving altitude sickness and reducing anxiety, hypertension, and blood pressure. Reishi preparations, widely used in China and Japan, are increasingly well-known in the West.

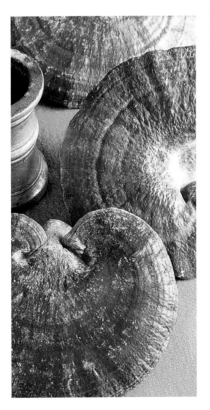

Used For:
Stimulating immunity • Calming anxiety • General tonic

Preparations:
Dried, powdered; capsules, extracts, tablets, tinctures.

Typical Dosages:
Capsules: Up to five 420 mg capsules a day.
Tablets: Up to three 1-gram tablets up to 3 times a day.
Or follow manufacturer's or practitioner's recommendations.

Cautions:
Experimental studies have shown toxicity is very low. Rare side effects after long-term use include dry throat, nosebleed, and upset stomach. Rare skin rashes have been reported as well as an allergic reaction in one patient who received an injectable form of the herb in China.

Rhubarb

Rheum palmatum and *R. officinale*

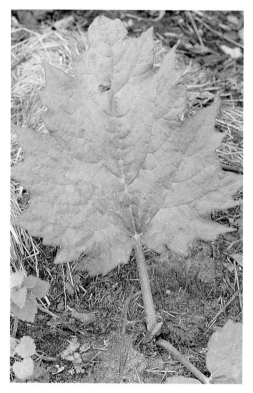

Sources: We are not talking about the rhubarb in your garden (*R. ×cultorum*), whose stems are used for pies and such. Rather, the subject of our discussion is the medicinal rhubarbs, with broad-lobed leaves, whose roots are a famous herbal laxative. Also known as Chinese, Turkey, or medicinal rhubarbs, *R. palmatum* and *R. officinale* are members of the buckwheat family. Most of the supply comes from China.

Traditional Use: The roots of medicinal rhubarb have been used as laxatives for at least 5,000 years. The herb originated in China and was imported into Europe in the first century A.D. when it was described by the Romans Dioscorides and Pliny. The thirteenth century Venetian explorer, Marco Polo, imported the root to Europe. It has been used as a laxative in China since 2700 B.C.

Current Use: The root is both astringent and laxative. Once the most valued laxative in the world, rhubarb root has been largely replaced by other natural or synthetic drugs. In small doses it is considered astringent and is used for diarrhea and stomachache. In larger doses it is strongly laxative and has been traditionally favored for use when hemorrhoids are present (due to the accompanying astringent effect). In the intestines, the anthroquinone glycosides in rhubarb are chemically converted by bacteria into active components that produce a stimulant laxative effect. In addition to inhibiting the uptake of water and electrolytes in the large intestine, these compounds also stimulate intestinal motility. Rhubarb root has also figured in herbal cleansing and slimming programs, in my opinion an inappropriate use of a legitimate laxative that should be used only as directed.

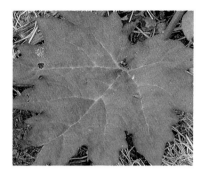

Used For:
Constipation

Preparations:
Dried root, whole, cut and sifted, powdered; included in herbal laxatives.

Typical Dosages:
As a stomach tonic, a pinch of finely chopped or powdered dried root. As a laxative, 1/3–1/2 teaspoon dried root.
Tea: Steep 1/3 tsp dried root in 1 cup hot water for 10–15 minutes. Do not take more than 2 times a day, and limit usage to a few days.
Tincture: 15–30 drops up to 4 times a day.
Or follow manufacturer's or practitioner's recommendations.

Cautions:
As with other stimulating plant-derived laxatives, rhubarb should be used only on a short-term basis. Laxative abuse can cause loss of potassium and other electrolytes, and pigmentation of the intestines. When laxatives have been abused and potassium lost, rhubarb root may increase the effects of cardiotonic glycosides. In cases of intestinal obstruction, avoid laxatives. Normal bowel function depends on a diet with plenty of fluids and roughage, along with exercise.

Rosemary

Rosmarinus officinalis

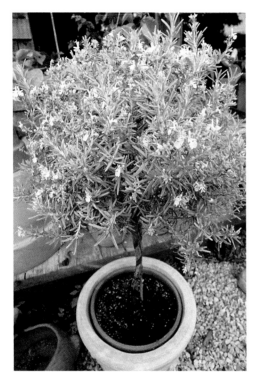

Sources: Rosemary is a culinary herb familiar to all. This relatively tender shrub in the mint family is native to the Mediterranean from Spain and Portugal south to Morocco and Tunisia. The leaves are harvested and dried. Some rosemary is produced commercially in the United States, but most is imported from the Mediterranean region.

Traditional Use: Shakespeare's Ophelia immortalized rosemary in the line from *Hamlet,* "There's rosemary, that's for remembrance." Indeed, in the ancient world, rosemary was thought to strengthen the memory and comfort the brain. In his 1653 *Complete Herbal,* the English herbalist Nicholas Culpeper observes, "It helpeth a weak memory and quickeneth the senses." Rosemary was official in the *United States Pharmacopoeia* from 1820 to 1950, valued primarily as a diuretic, an antispasmodic, an aromatic stimulant to digestion, and a treatment for menstrual difficulties. Externally, leaf preparations have been used for eczema and wounds that are slow to heal.

Current Use: In modern European phytomedicine, rosemary is valued for treating upset stomach, digestive gas, and a feeling of distention in the abdomen. It is also used as an appetite stimulant to promote gastric secretions. In Germany, rosemary is approved for use in dyspeptic complaints and rheumatism. For circulatory disorders, it is used as a counterirritant to stimulate blood circulation. The herb has antispasmodic and anti-inflammatory effects and stimulates increased coronary blood flow. It contains a number of potent antioxidant components, which has led to commercial use of isolated compounds and extracts as preservatives for processed foods. Free-radical-scavenging and liver-protecting activity comparable to milk thistle's have also been shown. Significant hyperglycemic and insulin release inhibitory effects have been identified for the essential oil in animal experiments. Several studies have shown that rosemary may help protect against development of tumors.

Used For:
Digestion • Rheumatism • Stimulating appetite • Stimulating circulation

Preparations:
Dried, whole leaf, powdered; tinctures, extracts. Leaf extracts in Europe are standardized to the antioxidant carnosol.

Typical Dosages:
Bath: Steep about 1¾ oz (50 g) in a full bath.
Tea: Steep 1 tsp dried leaf in 1 cup hot water for 10–15 minutes. Use up to 3 times a day.
Or follow manufacturer's or practitioner's recommendations.

Cautions:
Rosemary and its essential oil should be avoided during pregnancy because the herb may have adverse effects on the uterus or fetus. No side effects, contraindications, or drug interactions are reported for the leaves. The highly concentrated essential oil, however, can cause gastroenteritis or kidney damage. One case of dermatitis has been reported from exposure to a carnosol-standardized extract of rosemary during the manufacturing process. The herb is generally considered safe for flavoring food.

Sage

Salvia officinalis

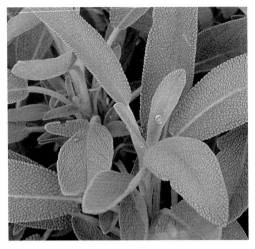

Sources: The common garden sage, *Salvia officinalis,* a member of the mint family, is best known as a culinary herb. This variable plant group is native to the Mediterranean, especially the Baltic region, with much of the commercial supply originating from wild-harvested plant material in Albania and the former Yugoslavia. There is also limited commercial production in the United States.

Traditional Use: The herb has been used both for culinary and medicinal purposes for more than 2,000 years. Traditionally an external folk medicine, the fresh, bruised leaves were applied to treat sprains, swellings, ulcers, and bleeding. The leaves were also used for

> **Pharmacological studies have confirmed sage's antibacterial, antifungal, antiviral, and astringent activities.**

rheumatic complaints, to reduce excessive menstrual bleeding and sweating, and to dry up a mother's milk. Like rosemary, sage was valued for its ability to improve memory and sharpen the senses. A sage gargle (often combined with rosemary and plantain) was used for sore throat and mouth and canker sores. Sage was official in the *United States Pharmacopoeia* from 1840 to 1900. General historical usage for dyspepsia and oral inflammations are the same as in modern times.

Current Use: In modern European phytomedicine, a gargle of sage tea is used to treat sore throat, inflammations of the mouth and mucous membranes, and as a mouthwash for gingivitis. Depending on dose, the tea is used internally to treat upset stomach, night sweats, and excessive sweating. Pharmacological studies have confirmed antibacterial, antifungal, antiviral, and astringent activities. Limited clinical studies have confirmed sweating inhibition. The potential health applications of sage have yet to be widely recognized.

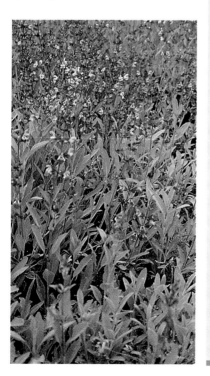

Used For:
Indigestion • Inflammation • Excessive sweating

Preparations:
Dried herb whole, ground, powdered; sometimes used in combination products.

Typical Dosages:
Tea: For upset stomach, steep 1 tsp dried herb in 1 cup hot water for 10–15 minutes. To reduce excessive sweating, use 2 tsp.
Tincture: 30–60 drops.
Or follow manufacturer's or practitioner's recommendations.

Cautions:
For medicinal purposes, sage should be used as needed in small amounts rather than taken over a long period of time. Like wormwood, sage and its essential oil and alcohol extracts contain thujone.

Prolonged use can result in dizziness, hot flashes, and seizures. Contact dermatitis is also reported from handling the herb. Proper identification is important, as a number of other sage species are common adulterants.

Sarsaparilla

Smilax spp.

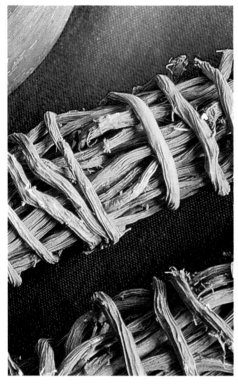

Sources: Sarsaparilla is the root of several South and Central American and Caribbean species of *Smilax,* a genus in the lily family. They include Mexican sarsaparilla (*S. medica,* also known as *S. aristolochiaefolia*), Honduran sarsaparilla (*S. regelii*), Ecuadorian sarsaparilla (*S. febrifuga*), Jamaican sarsaparilla (*S. ornata*), and other species. Most of the commercial supply is harvested from the wild.

Traditional Use: By 1530, Mexican sarsaparilla was exported to Europe to treat syphilis and rheumatism. It was an official treatment for syphilis in the *United States Pharmacopoeia* in 1850 and was often an ingredient in late nineteenth-century patent medicines promoted as blood purifiers, tonics, and diuretics and for a myriad of questionable applications. In recent years sarsaparilla has been touted as a male sexual rejuvenator with claims implying it contains testosterone. It has also been used as an anabolic-steroid replacement in natural bodybuilding formulas.

Current Use: Simply put, there is no credible recent research on the actions of sarsaparilla. A few studies in the 1930s and 1940s showed it to be diuretic, anti-inflammatory, and protective of the liver. Benefits were also claimed in cases of eczema and psoriasis. Sarsaparilla does contain plant steroids but nothing close to testosterone, because the body cannot convert plant steroids to anabolic steroids or human hormones. The collective scientific evidence, scarce as it is, shows that sarsaparilla is more likely to build profit margins than muscle tissue.

A number of species of *Smilax* are used in traditional Asian medical systems. Korean researchers have discovered new compounds, smilaxin A, B, and C, in Asian smilax or *S. sieboldii*. In animal studies, smilaxin B blocked nerves in the spinal column from sending pain signals to the brain. Its action was compared with that of opiates derived from opium poppies; smilaxin B worked in a different manner, but nevertheless had a significant effect. *S. sieboldii* is a likely subject for development as a painkiller.

Sarsaparilla extract is approved as a food flavoring ingredient in the United States. In Germany, where sarsaparilla has traditionally been used to treat skin diseases including psoriasis, as well as rheumatism and kidney ailments, products may not carry therapeutic claims because their effectiveness has not been demonstrated. After 500 years of use in the West, sarsaparilla still awaits careful studies.

Used For:
Flavoring

Preparations:
Dried root, powdered; capsules, tablets, tinctures, combination products.

Typical Dosages:
No therapeutic dosage has been established.
Capsules: Up to five 425 mg capsules a day.
Tea: Steep 1/2–2 tsp powdered root in 1 cup hot water for 10–15 minutes.
Tincture: 15–30 drops up to 3 times a day.
Or follow manufacturer's or practitioner's recommendations.

Cautions:
According to German health authorities, sarsaparilla preparations have caused stomach irritation and temporary kidney problems. Known to increase the absorption of digitalis and hasten the elimination of other medications, sarsaparilla should not be taken by anyone taking anything prescribed.

Saw Palmetto

Serenoa repens

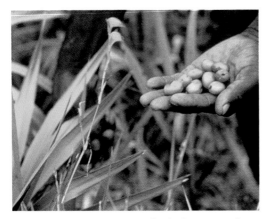

Source: Saw palmetto is the fruit of a small shrub in the palm family native to the southeastern United States. Most is wild-harvested in Florida.

Traditional Use: Saw palmetto was introduced into medicine by J. B. Read of Savannah, Georgia, in an 1879 issue of the *American Journal of Pharmacy:* "By its peculiar soothing power on the mucous membrane it induces sleep, relieves the most troublesome coughs, promotes expectoration, improves digestion, and increases fat, flesh, and strength. Its sedative and diuretic properties are remarkable."

An "original communication" in the July, 1892, issue of *The New Idea* stated, "It also exerts a great influence over the organs of reproduction, mammoa, ovarium, prostate, tests [sic], etc. Its action on them is a vitalizer, and is said to be the greatest known, tending to increase their activity and add greatly to their size."

Current Use: Clinical trials with saw palmetto show that it decreases symptoms associated with benign prostatic hyperplasia (BPH), especially the urge to urinate during the night. Fifty percent of men over fifty may develop BPH. Pressure of the enlarged prostate on the bladder may cause many of these men to awaken four or five times a night with the urge to urinate. Components of fat-soluble extracts in saw palmetto reduce prostate size and inhibit inflammation. A double-blind French clinical trial involving 110 BPH patients, published in 1984, reported that saw palmetto reduced the number of times that patients had to urinate at night by more than 45 percent and increased urinary flow by more than 50 percent. Painful or difficult urination was significantly reduced in the treatment group as compared to the placebo group.

A recent major study published in the journal *The Prostate* compared the use of Permixon, a European saw-palmetto extract, with the conventional drug finasteride (Proscar) in the treatment of 1,098 patients diagnosed with BPH. The researchers concluded that both treatments relieve symptoms of BPH in about two-thirds of patients. The conventional drug, finasteride, produced a significant decrease in prostate size but also decreased libido and potency. The saw palmetto product did not reduce prostate size, but produced fewer complaints of decreased libido or impotence. This study confirms that saw palmetto relieves symptoms of BPH while producing fewer side effects than the conventional drug.

German health authorities allow saw palmetto use for urinary difficulties in early stages of BPH.

Used For:
Benign prostatic hyperplasia (BPH)

Preparations:
Dried fruit whole, ground; capsules, tablets, tinctures. Standardized products made with fat-soluble carriers containing high levels of free fatty acids.

Typical Dosages:
Standardized preparations are taken one or two times a day for a daily dose of 320 mg. 1/2–1 tsp of the dried fruit is the average daily dose of other preparations.
Capsules (non-standardized): Up to three 585 mg capsules a day.
Tincture: 20–30 drops up to 4 times a day.
Or follow manufacturer's or practitioner's recommendations.

Cautions:
No side effects or contraindications other than rare stomach upset have been reported. BPH can only be diagnosed by a physician, who should be consulted for proper examination and treatment.

Schisandra

Schisandra chinensis

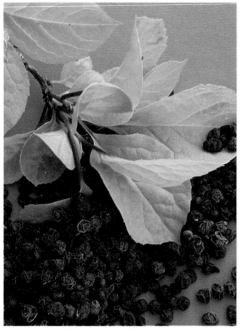

Sources: The genus *Schisandra* of the magnolia vine family includes about twenty-five species, all native to eastern Asia with the exception of *S. coccinea,* a rare vine of the southeastern United States. While *S. chinensis* is sometimes an ornamental vine in American gardens, the herb user is more likely to find its dried fruits in a Chinese herb shop or a health food store. The Chinese name *wu-wei-zi* means "five-flavor seeds" for the balanced taste that is sweet, sour, bitter, pungent (hot), and salty all at once. Most of the supply comes from China, though there is some production in eastern Europe and Russia.

Traditional Use: Listed in the primary class of herbs in *Shen Nong Ben Cao Jing* and an official remedy in the *Chinese Pharmacopoeia,* schisandra fruits are widely used in Traditional Chinese Medicine as a general tonic and for cough and nervous and liver conditions, uses confirmed by modern research.

Current Use: Schisandra's biological activity is primarily attributed to a group of compounds known as lignans (about 19 percent of the fruit weight). Like *Panax ginseng* and Siberian ginseng, schisandra is considered to be adaptogenic, but somewhat weaker and less toxic. Laboratory experiments coupled with clinical trials confirm that, in healthy individuals, schisandra helps to improve brain efficiency, increase work capacity, stimulate the central nervous system, improve reflexes, build strength, and increase endurance. Other studies have shown that schisandra helps to normalize blood pressure and is strongly antioxidant. Recent research has focused on the effect of schisandra preparations on the liver. Exhibiting a liver-protectant effect similar to milk thistle, schisandra is widely used in China to treat hepatitis or exposure to liver-toxic industrial chemicals. The herb has yet to make a strong impact in the American market, probably because most of the scientific research has been published in Chinese, Japanese, or Russian.

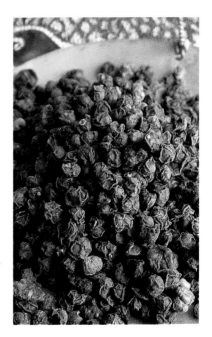

Used For:
Tonic • Liver protection • Antioxidant

Preparations:
Dried fruit, whole, powdered; capsules, tablets, tinctures, combination products.

Typical Dosages:
Capsules: Up to six 580 mg capsules a day.
Tea: Steep 1/3–1½ tsp dried fruit in 1 cup hot water for 10–15 minutes.
Tincture: 15–25 drops 2 times a day.
Or follow manufacturer's or practitioner's recommendations.

Cautions:
May cause gastrointestinal upset in some individuals.

Senna

Cassia acutifolia, C. senna

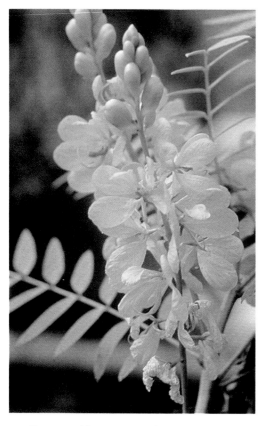

Sources: Senna is the dried leaf or pod of Alexandria senna and Tinnevelley senna. Both species have recently been referred to by botanists as *Senna alexandrina*. They are members of the pea family native to Eurasia and now cultivated commercially in the Middle East and India. Tinnevelley senna is used most frequently in the United States.

Traditional Use: Tea of the powdered senna leaf has been used for centuries, in both Eastern and Western traditions, for its laxative qualities.

Current Use: Senna does one thing, and does it well—relieve constipation. When senna is digested, it stimulates propulsive contractions and inhibits stationary contractions in the colon, thereby speeding elimination of waste and increasing water and electrolyte content.

Senna leaves contain about half as many active compounds as the pods, but they are considered safer to use. Senna is less expensive than cascara sagrada, but it is a stronger laxative with a greater tendency to cause cramping. The leaves, as well as the compounds extracted from them, are still official drugs in the *United States Pharmacopoeia*.

Used For:
Constipation

Preparations:
Dried leaf, pods; see cautions.

Typical Dosage:
Follow manufacturer's or practitioner's recommendations.

Cautions:
Senna should not be used for more than a week without a physician's advice. Longer use can make the bowels sluggish and bring about dependency on laxatives. Proper diet and exercise will do much to prevent the need for laxatives. Some individuals may experience discomfort or cramping after using senna products. In addition to sluggish bowel, prolonged use can lead to fluid and electrolyte imbalances, such as potassium loss, which can reduce the effectiveness of prescribed heart medications. Avoid using senna with licorice root, thiazide diuretics, or steroids because of the potential for potassium loss. Senna should not be used by pregnant or nursing women or children under ten years of age.

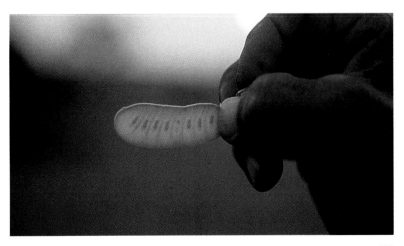

Shepherd's Purse

Capsella bursa-pastoris

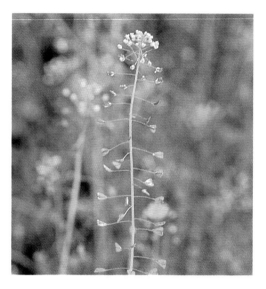

Sources: Shepherd's purse is a small annual member of the mustard family native to southern Europe and western Asia that has become established as a scattered weed in much of North America. It gets its common name from the likeness of the seed pods to an old-fashioned leather purse. The whole herb is harvested when in fruit. Most of the supply comes from Europe.

Traditional Use: Traditionally, herbalists have considered shepherd's purse to be one of the best herbs for stopping bleeding, both internally and externally. It has been used to allay bleeding in the stomach, lungs, uterus, and kidneys, where it is also valued for urinary antiseptic qualities.

> **Herbalists have considered shepherd's purse to be one of the best herbs for stopping bleeding, both internally and externally.**

Current Use: European phytomedicine employs shepherd's purse for treatment of menstrual bleeding, nosebleeds, and for bleeding wounds. Pharmacological studies have shown that the herb possesses anti-inflammatory, diuretic, and antiulcer activity, but no one component or compound group is primary. The whole herb produces the effects. It has also been shown to decrease blood pressure in laboratory animals, and hemostatic activity has also been confirmed. Studies have shown that both water and methanolic extracts of the herb accelerate blood coagulation. In Germany use is approved for mild cases of prolonged, excessive, or irregular menstrual bleeding as well as to stop nosebleed and bleeding from wounds. More research is needed on this valuable traditional remedy.

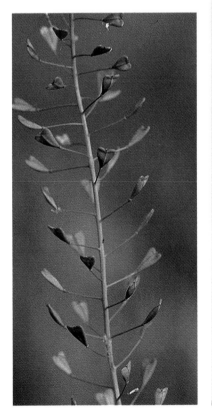

Used For:
Excessive bleeding

Preparations:
Whole dried herb, cut and sifted, powdered; capsules, tablets, tinctures.

Typical Dosages:
Tea: Steep 1–2 tsp dried herb in 1 cup hot water for 10–15 minutes. Use up to 3 times a day.
Tincture: 15–30 drops up to 3 times a day.
Or follow manufacturer's or practitioner's recommendations.

Cautions:
No contraindications or side effects are associated with this herb. Effects on uterine activity, hypertension, and hypotension are related to experimental injections of the herb, not oral medication. Since the herb can affect the uterus, safety dictates avoiding use during pregnancy.

Skullcap

Scutellaria lateriflora

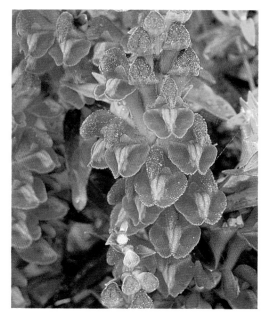

Source: Skullcap is a member of the mint family from the rich woods and moist soils of eastern North America. Another commonly used species is Baikal skullcap, (*S. baicalensis*), the root of which is the Chinese drug *huang-qin*. It is found in sandy fields in northeast China and adjacent Russia and in the mountains of southwest China.

Traditional Use: Also known as mad-dog skullcap, the American species has been used historically to treat rabies. Traditionally it is known as a nerve tonic and sedative for relieving anxiety, neuralgia, and insomnia. First mentioned in the middle class of drugs in *Shen Nong Ben Cao Jing,* Baikal skullcap is found in Chinese prescriptions for fevers, colds, high blood pressure, hypertension, insomnia, headache, intestinal inflammation, and vomiting of blood.

> **Also known as mad-dog skullcap, the American species has been used historically to treat rabies.**

Current Use: Almost all recent research has been done on Baikal skullcap. Numerous Chinese studies show that it inhibits bacteria and viruses, is diuretic, and lowers fevers and blood pressure; in China, it is also used to treat hepatitis. One of the few studies done on American skullcap has shown it to offer mild sedative and antispasmodic properties; this herb is a good candidate for further research.

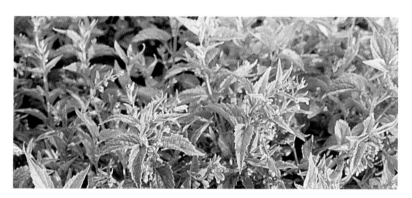

Used For:
Mild sedation

Preparations:
Dried herb; capsules, tablets, tea, tincture.

Typical Dosages:
Capsules: Up to six 425 mg capsules a day.
Tea: Steep 1–2 tsp dried herb in 1 cup hot water for 10–15 minutes.
Tincture: 20–40 drops up to 4 times a day.
Or follow manufacturer's or practitioner's recommendations.

Cautions:
American skullcap is often adulterated with *Teucrium canadense* traded as pink skullcap. The common garden germander, *T. chamaedrys*, has been linked to liver damage.

Slippery Elm
Ulmus rubra

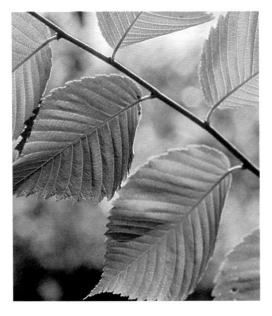

Sources: Slippery elm is the inner bark of a tree in the elm family, formerly known as *Ulmus fulva,* native from Maine through the St. Lawrence valley, west to the Dakotas, south to Texas, and east to Florida. To harvest it from wild trees, the rough outer bark is removed and the inner bark retained.

Traditional Use: Slippery elm was one of the most useful medicinal plants of the American wilderness. Native Americans from the Missouri River Valley used a tea of the fresh inner bark for a soothing laxative. Among the Creek, a poultice of the bark was a toothache remedy. The Osage and other groups applied bark poultices to extract thorns and gunshot balls. Surgeons during the American Revolution used bark poultices as their primary treatment for gunshot wounds, and a soldier, separated from his company, survived for ten days in the wilderness on the bark of slippery elm and sassafras. During the War of 1812, when food was scarce, British soldiers fed their horses on slippery elm bark. Nineteenth-century physicians recommended

> **Surgeons during the American Revolution used bark poultices as their primary treatment for gunshot wounds.**

slippery elm broth as a wholesome and nutritious food for infants and invalids, and the tea has long been the herbal treatment of choice for acute stomach ulcers and colitis. Adopted as an official drug for the first *United States Pharmacopoeia* in 1820, slippery elm was listed until 1936.

Current Use: Slippery elm is a good example of an herb that indisputably works well for a particular purpose. The inner bark contains high amounts of mucilage which, when mixed with water, soothe irritated mucous membranes of the the throat and intestinal tract. Slippery elm is still approved by the FDA as a nonprescription product for demulcent use.

Used For:
Gastrointestinal irritation • Sore throat

Preparations:
Dried bark, cut and sifted, powdered. There are few processors of slippery elm bark because it is highly combustible.

Typical Dosages:
Capsules: Up to twelve 370 mg capsules a day.
Tea: Steep 1/2 tsp powdered bark in a cup of hot water. Take 2–3 times a day.
Tincture: 10–30 drops up to 5 times a day.
Or follow manufacturer's or practitioner's recommendations.

Cautions:
No side effects or special cautions are noted.

St.-John's-Wort

Hypericum perforatum

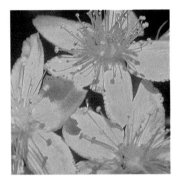

Source: St.-John's-wort is the dried herb or flowering top of a plant native to Europe and naturalized in Asia, Africa, North America, South America, and Australia. In 1793 the first recorded specimen in the United States was collected in Pennsylvania. Commercial supplies come from plants cultivated and wild-harvested in Chile, the United States, and Europe.

Traditional Use: St.-John's-wort has interested herbalists since the first-century Greek physicians Galen and Dioscorides recommended it as a diuretic, wound-healer, and treatment for menstrual disorders. During the Middle Ages, remarkable, even mystical properties were attributed to St.-John's-wort, thought to be best if harvested on June 24, St. John's Day. In nineteenth-century America, it was used by physicians for wound healing, especially for lacerations involving damaged nerves, and as a diuretic, astringent, and mild sedative.

Current Use: St.-John's-wort has emerged as the most popular herb in the United States, thanks to a segment aired June 27, 1997, on the ABC News program *20/20*. At least twenty-three controlled clinical studies involving more than 1,800 outpatients diagnosed with mild to moderate depression have been documented. In fifteen trials, St.-John's-wort preparations were compared with a placebo. Eight other trials compared St.-John's-wort to standard antidepressant drugs; six involved St.-John's-wort preparations and two used combination products. Fewer than 1 percent of patients in the trials dropped out because of side effects from St.-John's-wort, compared with 3 percent on standard drugs. Side effects have been reported in 19.8 percent of patients taking St.-John's-wort, while 52.8 percent experienced side effects with standard medications.

In a recent randomized, placebo-controlled, double-blind study of 105 outpatients diagnosed with mild to moderate depression or temporary depressive moods, 67 percent of those taking St.-John's-wort improved, but only 28 percent of the placebo group. Patients who took the St.-John's-wort felt significant improvement in depressive mood indicators such as feelings of sadness, hopelessness, helplessness, uselessness, fear, and difficult or disturbed sleep. No significant side effects were observed. Researchers conclude that, compared with synthetic antidepressants, St.-John's-wort extract produces side effects of minor significance and can be recommended for the treatment of mild and moderate depression.

Externally, St.-John's-wort oil is used for the treatment of wounds, abrasions, and first-degree burns.

Used For:
Mild to moderate depression • Cuts and abrasions (externally)

Preparations:
Dried herb, flowering tops for tea or soaked in oil for external use; capsules, tablets, tinctures. Most products for internal use are standardized to 0.2–0.3% hypericin. Standardized products may also include hyperoside, rutin, quercitin, cholorogenic acid.

Typical Dosages:
Capsules: For products standardized to 0.3% hypericin, take 300 mg 3 times a day.
Tea: Steep 1/2–1 tsp of dried herb (containing 0.2–1.0% hypericin) in a cup of hot water for 10–15 minutes.
Tincture: 15–40 drops up to 3 times a day.
Or follow manufacturer's or practitioner's recommendations.

Cautions:
Hypericin from the flowers may cause people with fair skin to break out in hives or blisters upon exposure to sunlight, a reaction called photodermatitis. If you are taking St.-John's-wort, stay out of the sun *and* the tanning salon! Yes, herbs are natural. So are deadly poisonous plants. Treat nature with respect.

Stinging Nettle

Urtica dioica

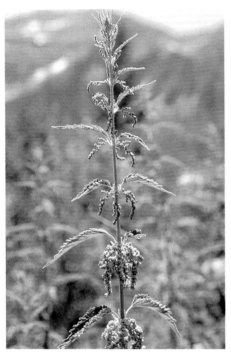

Sources: Stinging nettle is a perennial member of the nettle family, native to Europe and the United States. The root and leaf are used.

Traditional Use: In folk medicine, the dried herb and fresh plant juice have been used as diuretics, astringents, blood builders, and to treat anemia (nettle's iron content is high). The powdered leaves or fresh leaf juice have been applied to cuts to stop bleeding or taken in tea to treat excessive menstrual flow, nosebleeds, and hemorrhoids. Nettle tea has been used to stimulate circulation and as a spring tonic for chronic skin ailments. France's official bulletin on herbal medicines notes that it is traditionally used for the treatment of mild acne and eczema. It is also a folk treatment for arthritis.

Current Use: Recent studies suggest that nettle tea aids coagulation and formation of hemoglobin in red blood cells. A freeze-dried nettle-leaf product has shown slight activity in the treatment of allergies. Several studies indicate that the leaf extract depresses the central nervous system and inhibits bacteria and adrenaline. Stinging nettle's diuretic activity has been the subject of a number of German studies. Animals fed stinging nettle showed increased excretion of chlorides and urea. The juice has a distinctly diuretic effect in patients with heart disorders or chronic venous insufficiency. The herb's high levels of potassium and flavonoids may contribute to its diuretic action. In Germany, the herb is used for supportive treatment of rheumatic complaints and kidney infections.

Now stinging nettle root is attracting new research interest. German health authorities allow root preparations to be used for symptomatic relief of urinary difficulties associated with the early stages of benign prostatic hyperplasia (BPH). The root preparation increases urinary output and decreases the urge to urinate at night. Studies suggest that the root extract may inhibit interaction between a growth factor and its receptor in the prostate.

Researchers in New York recently examined the effect of various stinging nettle extracts to see if they had the ability to modulate sex-hormone binding globulins. They found that a water extract of stinging nettle was active in preventing the binding of SHBG to its receptor on prostatic membranes, whereas an alcohol extract of stinging nettle root was not active. This suggests that the compound responsible for biological activity in stinging nettle lies in a water soluble fraction, and provides clues on how the herb works in the treatment of benign prostatic hyperplasia.

Used For:
Benign prostatic hyperplasia (BPH) • Diuresis • Anemia

Preparations:
Dried leaf, dried root (combined with saw palmetto); capsules, tablets, tea, tincture.

Typical Dosages:
Capsules: Up to six 435 mg capsules a day.
Tea: Steep 1 tsp dried root in a cup of hot water and divide into 2 or 3 daily doses.
Or follow manufacturer's or practitioner's recommendations.

Cautions:
Fresh nettle leaves sting! The burning sensation usually lasts for about an hour but may persist for up to twelve hours in some individuals. No side effects or contraindications are reported for nettle products. The primary condition for which the roots are used, BPH, can be diagnosed only by a physician.

Tea Tree

Melaleuca alternifolia

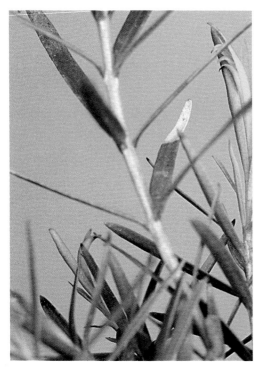

Sources: Tea tree is a small tree in the myrtle family that grows in wet ground on the northern coast of New South Wales and southern Queensland, Australia. The essential oil is produced commercially on plantations in New South Wales.

Traditional Use: Interest in tea tree oil emerged in the 1920s when Australian researchers found it had up to thirteen times more antiseptic activity than carbolic acid, then a well-known germicide. In 1930, *The Medicinal Journal of Australia* revealed that the oil, when applied to carbuncles and other infections, dissolved pus and inhibited bacterial growth without damaging surrounding tissues. Further studies established the oil as a disinfectant in soaps, a topical treatment for parasitic skin diseases, and a deodorant for wounds. A couple of drops in a glass of water were recommended as a gargle for sore throat at early stages of inflammation. Tea tree's confirmed antiseptic activity, gentleness to oral mucosa, and apparent lack of toxicity have endeared it to Australian dentists. Physicians use the oil to treat throat infections, dirty wounds, candida, and fungal infections like ring-worm and athlete's foot.

Current Use: Tea tree oil is now one of Australia's more popular herbal exports. A 1990 clinical trial involving 124 patients provides evidence of its effectiveness in the treatment of facial acne. In this study, a 5-percent solution of tea tree oil was slower to act than a conventional peroxide lotion, but caused less scaling, dryness, itching, and irritation.

A recent multicenter, randomized, double-blind clinical study of 117 patients has found that 100-percent tea tree oil is effective when applied topically to fungus-infected toenails. Another recent study has found that tea tree oil exhibits strong activity against antibiotic-resistant strains of bacteria.

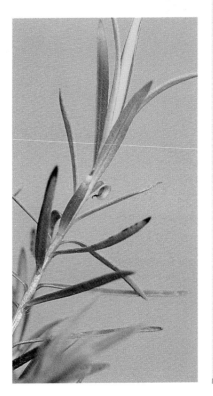

Used For:
Acne • Candida • Fungus

Preparations:
Essential oil, vaginal suppositories for candida. The Australian quality standard for tea tree oil is 30% terpinen-4-ol and less than 15% cineol.

Typical Dosage:
For external use only. Follow manufacturer's or practitioner's recommendations.

Cautions:
None noted, though as with all essential oils, some individuals may experience contact dermatitis. Internally, all essential oils are potentially toxic. Use only as directed.

Thyme

Thymus vulgaris

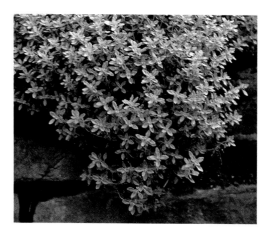

Sources: Thyme is a small shrub in the mint family native to the western Mediterranean region and southern Italy. The genus *Thymus* is represented by upwards of 300 species in temperate regions. Thyme is a well-known flavoring, often used for meat dishes and liquors. The name thyme is said to derived from the Greek word *thumus,* denoting courage which, in ancient times, the herb was considered to excite. Most thyme is imported from Europe, though some is produced in the United States.

Traditional Use: Thyme, both fresh and dried, is traditionally valued as an expellant for hookworms, a carminative for relieving digestive gas, an antispasmodic, mild sedative, expectorant, and means of inducing sweating in colds and fevers. It has long been employed for acute bronchitis, laryngitis, asthma, whooping cough, gastritis, diarrhea, and lack of appetite. Thyme baths have been used to help relieve rheumatic pains and promote healing of bruises and sprains. Both thyme herb and oil of thyme have been used in medicine. Oil of thyme is a highly concentrated, toxic compound.

Current Use: Studies conducted on the mechanism of thyme's action suggest that it eases bronchial spasms. Its active portion is the essential oil, composed largely of thymol and widely used as an antiseptic in the early part of this century. Today, German health authorities allow thyme to be labeled for "symptoms of bronchitis and whooping cough, and catarrhs of the upper airways."

Recently, Japanese researchers looked at the antioxidant potential of thyme. Among the compounds in the leaves they found a flavonoid and an extremely potent antioxidant. Both of these compounds had a strong ability to be effective in protecting biological systems against harmful oxidation processes and resulting tissue damage. These preliminary laboratory studies showed very promising results.

Bronchitis researchers in England and Germany recently reported on a controlled multi-center study comparing several herbal preparations with synthetic drugs. One product was a tablet containing dried extracts of primula root and thyme (*Thymus vulgaris*). This post-marketing surveillance study, conducted by 771 German physicians on 7,783 patients, found that the primula/thyme combination was equal to synthetic drugs in effectiveness, and more effective in adults.

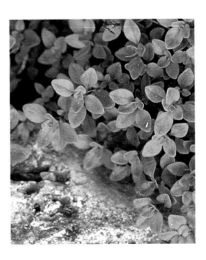

Used For:
Bronchitis • Whooping cough • Catarrh

Preparations:
Whole herb, cut and sifted, powdered. In Europe, available as thyme oil, thyme syrup, lozenges, fresh juice; capsules, tablets, tinctures.

Typical Dosage:
Tea: Steep 1 tsp dried herb in 1 cup hot water for 10–15 minutes. Use up to 4 times a day. Or follow manufacturer's or practitioner's recommendations.

Cautions:
Generally speaking, thyme herb is free from side effects, with no known contraindications or drug interactions. However, thyme essential oil can be toxic even in relatively small doses, irritating both the skin and mucous membranes.

Turmeric

Curcuma longa (syn. *C. domestica*)

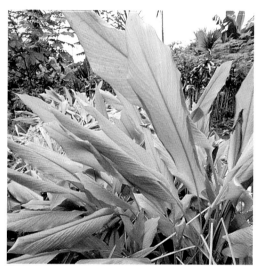

Sources: Long recognized as an important spice and dye plant, turmeric has recently emerged as an important medicinal herb as well. This tropical member of the ginger family continues to grow in popularity. Most of the supply comes from tropical Asian countries.

Traditional Use: In Thailand, turmeric rhizomes have been used to treat dizziness, gonorrhea, and peptic ulcers and as an appetite stimulant, carminative, astringent, and antidiarrheal. Externally, the rhizome is used to treat insect bites, ringworm, wounds, bleeding, and the teeth and gums. In Thailand, turmeric is one of the most important folk remedies, with official sanction for use. In India, it is used as a digestive aid, tonic, blood purifier, and antispasmodic. Among the herbs often classified as spices, turmeric is one of the best-researched for pharmacological effects.

Current Use: The typical yellow-orange color of turmeric comes from a yellow pigment found in the rhizomes called curcumin. Dietary supplements standardized to curcumin are now available in the market. Various studies have shown that curcumin possesses a number of important effects, including antioxidant, anti-inflammatory, cholesterol-lowering, and anticarcinogenic activity; specific complaints for which turmeric has been shown effective include peptic ulcers, atherosclerosis, and alcohol-induced liver toxicity. In one clinical study of smokers, curcumin was found to reduce the incidence of cell mutation. The anti-inflammatory activity of turmeric root has been compared to that of topical hydrocortisone.

It has also been shown to be of value for treatment of rheumatoid arthritis.

Turmeric is approved by German health authorities for the treatment of dyspeptic complaints, primarily because it stimulates secretion of bile from the gallbladder.

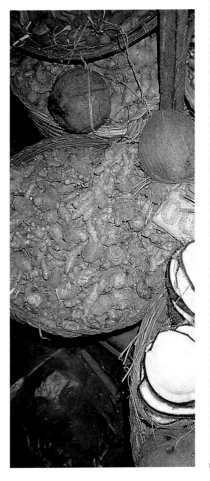

Used For:
Reducing inflammation • Indigestion • Antioxidant • Liver problems

Preparations:
Dried root, whole, powdered. Often standardized to up to 90% curcumin.

Typical Dosages:
Capsules (standardized): 250–500 mg up to 3 times a day.
Spice: Use up to 1 tsp a day in food.
Tincture: 10–30 drops up to 3 times a day.
Or follow manufacturer's or practitioner's recommendations.

Cautions:
No side effects or contraindications are generally reported. Use of the herb is contraindicated in cases of obstructions of the bile ducts; it should be used under medical supervision if gallstones are present.

Valerian

Valeriana officinalis

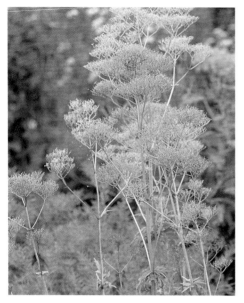

Sources: Valerian is the root of a perennial member of the valerian family found in eastern, southeastern, and east-central Europe, south Sweden, and the southern Alps. It escaped from cultivation in the northeastern United States and is commercially grown in Europe, the United States, and elsewhere.

Traditional Use: Valerian was best known to ancient classical authors as a diuretic and treatment for menstrual difficulties. The Greek physician Galen used it for epilepsy in children and adults. An Italian nobleman, Fabio Colonna, born in 1567, suffered from epilepsy and found Galen's reference. He took valerian himself and claimed it completely restored his health. Colonna's experience stimulated interest in the plant as a sedative; use of valerian to relieve spasms and induce sleep evolved in the seventeenth and eighteenth centuries. Valerian was an official remedy in the *United States Pharmacopoeia* from 1820 to 1936.

Current Use: Valerian is widely used in Europe as a mild sedative and sleep aid in cases of insomnia, excitability, and exhaustion. Experimental studies have shown that it depresses the central nervous system and relieves muscle spasms. Its sedative action is attributed to a number of chemical fractions, with no single compound emerging as the active principal.

In the 1980s Swiss researchers studied the effects of valerian water extracts on sleep patterns and found that valerian reduces the time taken to fall asleep, especially in older patients and insomniacs. Dream recall and nocturnal movement were apparently not affected, and no hangover effect, a common complaint among users of synthetic sedatives, was reported.

Ten controlled clinical studies have been published on valerian preparations, one of which suggests that valerian should be used for two to four weeks before daily mood and sleep patterns improve. The herb is therefore probably not appropriate for acute sleep disturbances.

German health authorities allow use of valerian in sedative and sleep-inducing preparations for states of excitation and for difficulty in falling asleep due to nervousness.

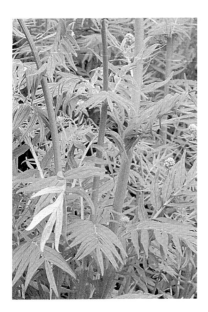

Used For:
Anxiety • Insomnia

Preparations:
Dried root, cut and sifted, powdered; tea, capsules, tablets, tinctures, extracts. Sometimes standardized to contain at least 0.5% essential oil.

Typical Dosages:
Capsules: For products standardized to 0.5% essential oil, take 300–400 mg a day. As a sleep aid, take 1 hour before bedtime.
Tincture: 20–60 drops a day.
Or follow manufacturer's or practitioner's recommendations.

Cautions:
Some individuals may experience temporary stomach upset. Compounds called valepotriates have been shown to destroy cells and cause mutations. Despite these findings, valerian is generally considered safe. Although official texts do not caution against using valerian during pregnancy, avoid it to be on the safe side.

Vitex

Vitex agnus-castus

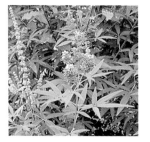

Sources: Vitex, or chaste tree, is the fruit of a shrub in the verbena family native to west Asia and southwestern Europe. It was introduced to Europe at an early date and is naturalized in much of the southeastern United States. The fruits are grown commercially in Europe.

Traditional Use: Vitex has been used for menstrual difficulties for at least 2,500 years. Hippocrates (460–377 B.C.) wrote, "If blood flows from the womb, let the woman drink dark wine in which the leaves of the vitex have been steeped." Its use for gynecological conditions is also noted in the works of Pliny (A.D. 23–79): "The trees furnish medicines that promote urine and menstruation." In the late 1800s, American physicians used a tincture of the fresh berries to increase milk secretion and treat menstrual disorders.

Current Use: During the past forty years, research has focused on the use of vitex for premenstrual syndrome (PMS) and menstrual difficulties. The biological activity cannot be attributed to a single chemical ingredient, though flavonoids are major components.

Between 5 and 30 percent of women may be affected by PMS. A 1992 survey of German gynecologists evaluated the effect of a vitex preparation on 1,542 women diagnosed with PMS. Both physicians and patients assessed effectiveness, with 90 percent reporting relief of symptoms after treatment averaging 25.3 days.

In a clinical study on the effectiveness and safety of long-term treatment with a vitex fruit tincture, 1,571 women with menstrual disorders and PMS were followed for a period of 7 days to 6 years (average 147.6 days). In 90 percent of patients, the treatment eliminated or alleviated symptoms of PMS.

Most studies have involved a tincture of the fruits. A recent study compared the efficacy of a tablet with the tincture in 175 women, and found that those who received 3.5 to 4.2 mg of dried extract of the fruit a day had a marked reduction of PMS symptoms such as breast tenderness, edema, tension, headache, constipation, and depression. It was found useful in 80 percent of the women and results were rated by practitioners as excellent in over 24 percent of cases. Twelve patients in this group reported gastrointestinal complaints, headaches, or mild skin reactions. These adverse effects were transient in nature. No serious side effects were observed. The researchers concluded that the dried berry extract of vitex was safe and effective in the treatment of PMS.

German health authorities allow vitex preparations for disorders of the menstrual cycle, pressure and swelling in the breasts, and PMS. In Germany, vitex preparations are frequently used in the safe and effective treatment of PMS, heavy or too-frequent periods, acyclic bleeding, infertility, suppressed menses, and other conditions. Vitex is an excellent example of an herbal medicine which serves as a low-priced tool in European gynecological practice, rather than as an "alternative" to conventional medical treatment.

Used For:
Menopausal difficulties • Menstrual difficulties • PMS

Preparations:
Dried fruit, whole, pulverized; capsules, tinctures, tablets, and combination products. Clinical studies in Europe were done on a proprietary extract and capsules called Agnolyt.

Typical Dosages:
Capsules (non-standardized): Up to three 650 mg capsules a day.
Tea: Steep 1 scant tsp dried, ground berries in 1 cup hot water for 10–15 minutes.
Tincture: 15–40 drops as directed.
Or follow manufacturer's or practitioner's recommendations.

Cautions:
Do not use vitex if you are pregnant or receiving hormone-replacement therapy. Rare side effects include early menstruation following delivery as well as rare cases of itching, rashes, and gastrointestinal symptoms. In clinical trials, side effects have been reported in fewer than 2 percent of patients.

White Oak

Quercus alba

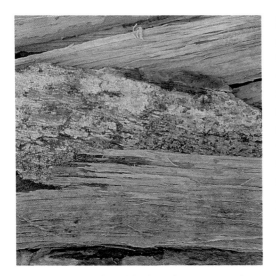

Sources: *Quercus* is the classical name of the oak tree, represented by over 400 species, primarily from the northern hemisphere, occurring as far south as the mountains of Colombia and Malaysia. More than seventy species and varieties are from Amcrican forests. Two basic groups are recognized in North America, the white oak group, (sub-genus *Leucobalanus*), and the red or black oak group (sub-genus *Erythrobalanus*). White oak grows from southern Maine to northern Florida, west to Texas, and northward through southeastern Kansas to Ontario and southwestern Quebec. The inner bark is used medicinally, and the supply is wild-harvested in eastern North America.

> **European settlers used white oak bark as a gargle for sore throats and an external wash for skin ailments.**

Traditional Use: Native Americans used white oak acorns as a food staple and the inner bark as an ingredient in cough medicine, as a tonic, an expectorant, and a treatment for rheumatism, bleeding hemorrhoids, diarrhea, dysentery, and wounds. In addition to these uses, European settlers used white oak bark as a gargle for sore throats and an external wash for skin ailments. White oak was listed in the *United States Pharmacopoeia* from 1820 until 1916, and in the *National Formulary* from 1916 to 1936.

Current Use: Very little scientific research has been conducted on white oak bark. The substances responsible for oak's powerful astringency are tannic acids; the astringency results from tannin's ability to precipitate proteins. Their biological activity includes antibacterial, antiviral, anticancer, cavity-stabilizing, and growth-depressant properties. In Germany, a related species, *Quercus robur,* is allowed externally for inflammatory skin disease and internally for diarrhea.

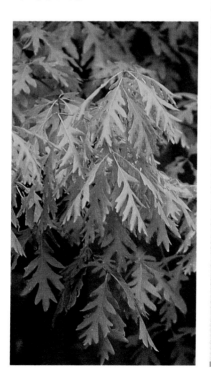

Used For:
Diarrhea • Reducing inflammation

Preparations:
Dried inner bark, whole, cut and sifted, powdered; capsules, formulations, tinctures.

Typical Dosages:
Capsules: Up to six 380 mg capsules a day.
Tea: Steep 1 tsp dried inner bark in 1 cup hot water for 10–15 minutes. Can also be used as a gargle or rinse for mouth inflammations.
Or follow manufacturer's or practitioner's recommendations.

Cautions:
In high concentrations, tannins can be carcinogenic, inhibiting the absorption of alkaloids. Gastric irritation, nausea, vomiting, and fatal liver damage have resulted from ingestion of large doses of tannins. White oak should be used only as needed and not on any regular basis as a dietary supplement.

Wild Yam

Dioscorea villosa

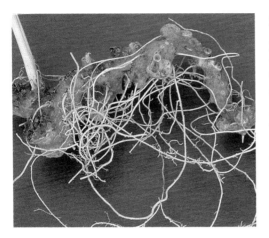

Sources: The genus *Dioscorea,* whose name honors the Roman physician and naturalist Dioscorides, is a large plant group with 850 species of warm temperate and moist tropical tuberous vines. *Dioscorea* species have been domesticated for their starchy roots throughout the world. In the United States, the common wild yam is found in moist woods from Connecticut south to Tennessee, west to Texas, and north to Minnesota. The root is wild-harvested. Mexican species also appear in the American market, often as wild yam or Mexican yam.

Traditional Use: Historically, wild yam was offered under the name "colic root" and used in Eclectic medical traditions for treating gastrointestinal problems such as irritation of the digestive tract, morning sickness, and "chronic gastritis of drunkards," as well as asthma and rheumatism. It was considered antispasmodic and anodyne by the Eclectics. Native American groups used the root to relieve labor pains. The traditional uses for rheumatism and childbirth suggest the possibility of estrogenic activity.

Current Use: Wild yam has reappeared in the American market in recent years as a "source" of estrogen and progesterone. Some have called this the "wild yam scam." Wild yam contains a compound called diosgenin, which was used as a starting material in early steroidal drugs, including birth-control pills. At one point, monopolistic Mexican sources of diosgenin increased the root's price sixfold, motivating drug manufacturers to switch to other plant sources for synthesizing the drugs.

In the 1990s, newspaper articles about wild yam made the erroneous claim that the body can transform diosgenin into steroid or hormone-like compounds. There is no reliable scientific evidence to suggest this is true. It has also been said that diosgenin is a natural source for the precursor for steroidal hormones, DHEA (dehydroepiandrosterone), itself a well-known dietary supplement. A recent clinical study involving seven healthy volunteers found that blood levels of DHEA did not increase after taking Mexican yam for three weeks. However, the yam did lower serum cholesterol levels. Antioxidant activity has also been ascribed to wild yam.

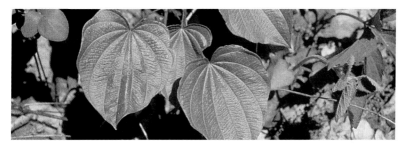

Used For:
Gastrointestinal problems

Preparations:
Dried tuber, whole, cut and sifted, powdered; capsules, topical products.

Typical Dosages:
No therapeutic dosage has been established.
Capsules: Up to two 405 mg capsules a day.
Tincture: 20–40 drops up to 5 times a day.
Or follow manufacturer's or practitioner's recommendations.

Cautions:
Some consumers report gastrointestinal irritation or upset from wild yam preparations. Some pharmacologic studies suggest that certain wild yam species may increase the time it takes blood to coagulate.

Willow

Salix spp.

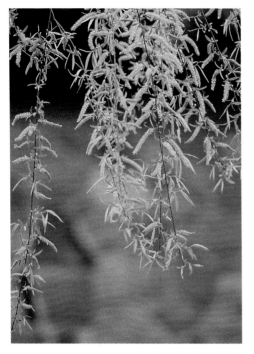

Sources: Willow is the inner bark of several species of *Salix,* trees in the willow family, including white willow (*S. alba*), crack willow (*S. fragilis*), purple willow (*S. purpurea*), violet willow (*S. daphnoides*), and bay willow (*S. pentandra*). All but bay willow are naturalized in North America.

Traditional Use: For more than 2,000 years, people of the northern hemisphere used willow bark as a wash for external ulcers and internally to reduce fevers and relieve aches, pains, rheumatism, arthritis, and headaches. The Houma used black willow root bark as a blood thinner; the Creek used the root tea to relieve inflammation in rheumatism and reduce fever. In American folk tradition, the bark was used to thin the blood and treat fever. The tea was also taken for dyspepsia. In 1763, a Dr. Stone of London first recommended willow bark to the medical profession for the treatment of fevers.

Current Use: In the 1890s the Bayer Company was looking for a substitute for wintergreen and black birch oil, then used to relieve pain, because the substances were simply too toxic. While studying experiments from 1853 in which salicylic acid was first synthesized from carbolic acid, Bayer researchers synthesized a derivative, acetylsalicylic acid, commonly known today as aspirin. No other drug is as well-known for its analgesic, fever-reducing, or anti-inflammatory qualities. Willow bark is considered a "natural aspirin."

Willow bark compounds are oxidized in the liver and blood to produce salicylic acid. It has pain-relieving effects like aspirin, but with fewer side effects. But can you take enough willow bark to achieve the effect of aspirin? According to Varro Tyler, probably not.

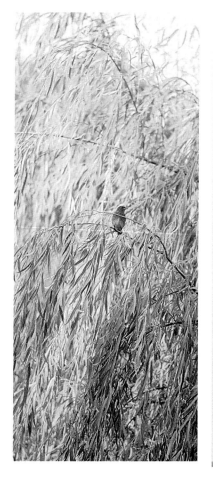

Used For:
Aches and pains • Fever

Preparations:
Dried bark, whole, cut and sifted, powdered; capsules, tablets, tea. European products are standardized to 1% salicin.

Typical Dosages:
Capsules: Up to six 400 mg capsules a day.
Tea: Steep 1/4–1/2 tsp powdered bark in 1 cup hot water for 10–15 minutes. Taken 3 times a day, this might not deliver more than 120 mg salicin—far less than a dose of aspirin.
Or follow manufacturer's or practitioner's recommendations.

Cautions:
Willow bark is high in tannins, which can damage the liver. Because willow bark produces salicin, it is contraindicated in the same instances as aspirin for stomach ulcers and, in children, for high fever.

Witch Hazel

Hamamelis virginiana

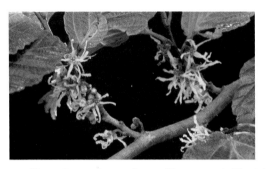

Sources: The common witch hazel, whose twigs, branches, bark, and leaves are used to make witch-hazel extracts, is a small shrub that flowers late, after the leaves have dropped, and is native from Nova Scotia west to Ontario and south to Texas and Florida. The genus *Hamamelis* includes five or six species found only in eastern North America and eastern Asia.

Traditional Use: Native peoples throughout eastern North America used witch hazel for a wide range of applications. Externally, it was used to treat rheumatism, relieve sore muscles, backache, cuts, bruises, insect bites, ulcers, tumors, sores, eye inflammations, and hemorrhoids. In the 1840s, Theron T. Pond of Utica, New York, learned from an Oneida healer that the shrub was held in high esteem for all types of burns, boils, and wounds. In 1848, Pond marketed an extract under the trade name "Golden Treasure." After several moves and sales, a manufacturing facility was established in Connecticut, and the name of the preparation was changed to "Pond's Extract." The witch-hazel industry is still centered in Connecticut where three manufacturers produce most of the witch-hazel extract sold on the American market.

Current Use: Witch hazel is an approved over-the-counter astringent for skin protection and relief of hemorrhoids. It contains various flavonoids, tannins, small amounts of volatile oil, and other components, which may be responsible for its astringent and hemostatic properties. Antioxidant, radiation-protective, and anti-inflammatory activity have been confirmed. A recent study found that witch hazel distillate, despite its anti-inflammatory activity, was not clinically useful (compared with hydrocortisone) for atopic eczema.

A Japanese research group initially screened extracts of sixty-five plants for their potential antioxidant activity. Seven were found promising and were selected for further research as possible antioxidant agents. The purpose of the study was to find plant compounds that protected cells in skin tissue from damage by harmful forms of oxygen. Of the seven plants tested, witch hazel and horse chestnut were found to have strong activity against reactive oxygen in skin tissue. The scientists proposed that both extracts be further researched for their potential use in antiaging or antiwrinkling skin products.

For more than 150 years, witch hazel has been valued for its for astringent, tonic, and mild pain-relieving qualities, used in treating hemorrhoids, itching, irritations, and other minor pains. Products include suppositories, cloth wipes, ointments, and lotions.

In Germany, witch hazel is approved for the treatment of mild diarrhea, inflammation of the gums and mucous membranes of the mouth, and mild irritation or local inflammation of the skin, hemorrhoids, and varicose veins.

Used For:
Skin irritation or mild inflammation • Mild diarrhea • Hemorrhoids

Preparations:
Distillate of stems and branches (witch-hazel water); dried leaves and bark, whole, cut and sifted, powdered.

Typical Dosage:
Tea: For internal use, steep 1 tsp bark (or 4 tsp dried leaves) in 1 cup hot water for 10–15 minutes. For external use, follow manufacturer's or practitioner's recommendations.

Cautions:
None are noted for topical preparations of the leaf or bark. Internally, stomach upset or irritation of the gastrointestinal tract has been reported. Tannins, in excess, may cause liver damage.

Yellow Dock

Rumex crispus

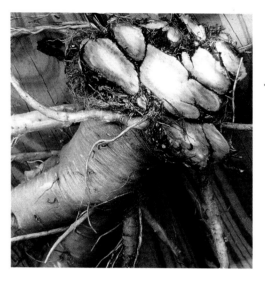

Sources: Yellow dock, a member of the buckwheat family, is native to Europe but widely naturalized throughout much of North America. The root is used in herbal traditions; the young leaves are sometimes used as wild greens. Most of the supply comes from Europe, though some root is commercially harvested from the wild or cultivated in North America.

Traditional Use: Yellow dock is historically considered a blood purifier, tonic, and mild astringent used to treat "bad blood," enlarged lymph nodes, skin conditions, nervous dyspepsia, and respiratory infections. The fresh, bruised root has been used externally for skin conditions. In nineteenth-century America, the root was prescribed for chronic skin diseases such as psoriasis, glandular deficiencies, jaundice, and constipation. A famous Shoshone medicine man, Rolling Thunder, thought highly of the herb; he called it "poor man's ginseng." Related species of common sorrel and sheep sorrel were considered useful as anti-inflammatories and folk cancer remedies. Sheep sorrel is one of the ingredients in the anticancer formula known as ESSIAC.

> **Yellow dock is historically considered a blood purifier, tonic, and mild astringent.**

Current Use: Anthraquinones, tannins, and oxalic acid have been identified from the roots, along with small amounts of an essential oil. There is no current pharmacological or clinical research on yellow dock.

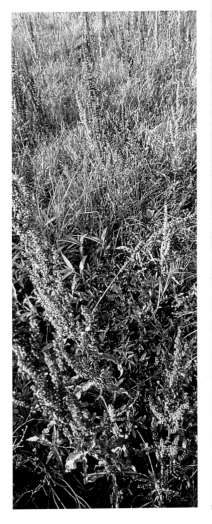

Used For:
Folk cancer remedy

Preparations:
Dried root, whole, cut and sifted, powdered; capsules, tincture.

Typical Dosages:
No therapeutic dosages have been established.
Capsules: Up to four 500 mg capsules a day.
Tincture: 20–40 drops up to 2 times a day.
Or follow manufacturer's or practitioner's recommendations.

Cautions:
Though considered slight, a laxative effect has been attributed to anthraquinones in yellow dock root, so it should be used only on a short-term basis. Oxalic acid content may result in disturbance of calcium metabolism. Avoid during pregnancy.

Yucca

Yucca schidigera

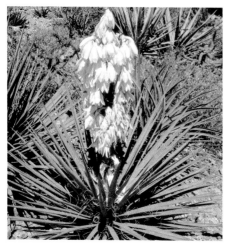

Sources: The genus *Yucca* in the agave family contains about thirty species native to warm regions of North America. The supply is primarily wild harvested from the desert southwest. The most commonly used species include *Y. schidigera, Y. brevifolia, Y. glauca,* and *Y. filamentosa,* among others. Most products in the market list *Y. schidigera* on the product label.

Traditional Use: *Yucca filamentosa,* also known as Adam's needle or bear grass, was used by the Cherokee to treat diabetes and sores and to reduce fevers. *Y. glauca,* also known as bear grass or soap weed, was used by Native Americans as a wash to make hair grow and externally to stop bleeding and reduce inflammation. Yuccas leaves were widely used for fiber, the roots for making soap and stunning fish. In Western herbal traditions, yucca roots have been valued for the treatment of diabetes, arthritis, and digestive disorders.

Current Use: Saponins in yucca roots are considered responsible for biological activity. A recent study found that extracts of *Y. schidigera,* added to cat and dog food, greatly reduced fecal odor, as determined by a panel of human sniffers. The poultry industry has looked at yucca extract as a feed additive to fatten chickens and turkeys. The results were mixed. A protein in *Y. recurvifolia* was found to have strong inhibitory activity against *Herpes simplex* virus. A polysaccharide fraction with antitumor activity has been identified from the fresh flowers of *Y. glauca.* Anti-inflammatory activity has been observed in a number of animal models. An extract of *Y. schidigera* was also found to have antimutagenic activity in a recent laboratory study. Antifungal, antitumor, and antiarthritic activity have been suggested by research.

Controversial clinical studies published in 1975 and 1978 issues of the *Journal of Applied Nutrition* suggested that a yucca extract was safe and effective for treating the pain, swelling, and stiffness of arthritic conditions. A follow-up study showed a reduction in blood pressure and cholesterol levels in a clinical study involving 212 patients. The studies subsequently deemed poorly controlled and the results were inconsistent. Despite these findings, the studies have led to widespread herbal use of yucca preparations for arthritic conditions. Yucca's bioactive compounds require further research.

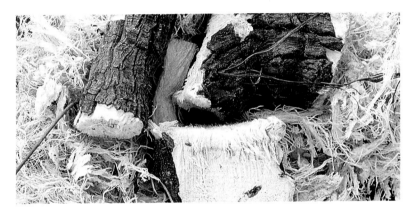

Used For:
Arthritis

Preparations:
Dried root, whole, cut and sifted, powdered; capsules.

Typical Dosage:
Capsules: Up to four 490 mg capsules a day.
Or follow manufacturer's or practitioner's recommendations.

Cautions
Yucca is not generally associated with toxicity, but should be used in moderation because little research has been done.

Bibliography

Herb References

Alfalfa

Bradley, B. A. 1915. "Uses of Alfalfa." In *Observation with* Medicago Sativa. Cincinnati: Lloyd Brothers.

Olin, B. R. (Ed.). 1991. "Alfalfa." *Lawrence Review of Natural Products* March:1–2.

Aloe Vera

Grindlay, D., and T. Reynolds. 1986. "The *Aloe vera* Phenomenon: A Review of the Properties and Modern Uses of the Leaf Parenchyma Gel." *Journal of Ethnopharmacology* 16:117–51.

Heggers, J. P. et al. 1995. "Wound-Healing Effects of *Aloe* Gel and Other Topical Antibacterial Agents on Rat Skin." *Phytotherapy Research* 9:455–57.

Heggers, J. P., R. P Pelley, and M. C. Robson. 1993. "Beneficial Effects of *Aloe* in Wound Healing." *Phytotherapy Research* 7: S48–S52.

Koo, M. W. L. 1994. "*Aloe vera:* Antiulcer and Anti-Diabetic Effects." *Phytotherapy Research* 8:461–64.

Leung, A. 1985. "*Aloe vera* Update: A New Form Questions Integrity of Old." *Drug & Cosmetic Industry* September:42–46.

Saito, H. 1993. "Purification of Active Substances of *Aloe arborescens* Miller and Their Biological and Pharmacological Activity." *Phytotherapy Research* 7:S14–S19.

Yongchaiyudha, S. et al. 1996. "Anti-Diabetic Activity of *Aloe vera* L. Juice. 1. Clinical Trial in New Cases of Diabetes Mellitus." *Phytomedicine* 3:241–43.

Arnica

ESCOP. 1997. *Arnicae Flos.* In *ESCOP Monographs on the Medicinal Use of Plant Drugs* (Vol. 4). Exeter, England: ESCOP Secretariat.

Ashwaganda

Atal, C. K. and A. E. Schwarting. 1961. "Ashawagandah—An Ancient Indian Drug." *Economic Botany* 15(3):256–63.

Bhattacharya, S. K., A. Kumar, and S. Ghosal. 1995. "Effects of Glycowithanolides from *Withania somnifera* on an Animal Model of Alzheimer's Disease and Perturbed Central Cholinergic Markers of Congition in Rats." *Phytotherapy Research* 9:110–13.

Grandhi, A., A. M. Mujumdar, and B. Patwardhan. 1994. "A Comparative Pharmacological Investigation of Ashwagandha and Ginseng." *Journal of Ethnopharmacology* 44:131–35.

Astragalus

Chu, D. A., et al. 1988. "Immunotherapy with Chinese Medicinal Herbs II. Reversal of Vyclphophamide-Induced Immune Suppression by Administration of Fractionated *Astragalus membranaceus in vivo.*" *Journal of Clinical and Laboratory Immunology* (1988):125–29.

Ros, L. and P. G. Waterman. 1997. "A Review of the Pharmacology and Toxicology of *Astragalus.*" *Phytotherapy Research* 11:411–18.

Sun, Y. et al. 1983. "Immune Restoration and/or Augmentation of Local Graft-Versus-Host Reaction by Traditional Chinese Medicine Herbs." 1983. *Cancer* 52(1):70–73.

Bearberry

ESCOP. 1997. *"Uvae ursi folium."* In *ESCOP Monographs on the Medicinal Use of Plant Drugs* (Vol. 5). Exeter, England: ESCOP Secretariat.

Bilberry

Bettini, V. et. al. 1984. "Effects of *Vaccinium myrtillus* Anthocanoside on Vascular Smooth Muscle." *Fitoterapia* 55(5): 265–272.

Bomser, J., et al. 1996. "*In vitro* Anticancer Activity of Fruit Extracts from *Vaccinium* Species." *Planta Medica* 62(3):212–16.

Cunio, L. 1993. "*Vaccinium myrtillus.*" *Australian Journal of Medical Herbalism* 5(4): 81–85.

Lietti, A. and G. Forni. 1976. "Studies of *Vaccinium myrtillus* Anthocanosides. I. Vasoprotective and Anti-Inflammatory

Activity." *Arnzeimittel Forschung-Drug Research* 26:829–32.

Black Cohosh

Beuscher, N. 1995. "*Cimicifuga racemosa* L.—Black cohosh." *Zeitschrift für Phytotherapie* 16:301–10.

Duker, E. M. et al. 1991. Effects of Extracts from *Cimicifuga racemosa* on Gonadotropin Release in Menopausal Women and Ovariectomized Rats." *Planta Medica* 57:420–24.

Foster, S. 1998. "Black cohosh—*Cimicifuga racemosa.*" *Botanical Series* no. 315. Austin: American Botanical Council.

Jarry, H., G. Harnischfeger and E. Dker. 1985. "Studies on the Endocrine Efficacy of the Constitutents of *Cimicifuga racemosa.* 2. *In vitro* Binding of Constituents to Estrogen Receptors." *Planta Medica* 51(4):316–19.

Lehmann-Willenbrock, E. and H. H. Riedel. 1988. Clinical and Endocrinological Examinations Concerning Therapy of Climacteric Symptoms Following Hysterectomy with Remaining Ovaries." *Zentralblatt für Gynakologie* 110(10):611–18.

Blessed Thistle

Vanhaelen-Fastre, R. 1973. "Constitution and Antibiotic Properties of the Essential Oil of *Cnicus benedictus.*" *Planta Medica* 24(2):165–75. (in French)

Zeller, W. M. de Gols and B. M. Hausen. 1985. "The Sensitizing Capacity of Compositae Plants. VI. Guinea Pig Sensitization Experiments with Ornamental Plants and Weeds Using Different Methods." *Archives of Dermatological Research* 277(1):28–35.

Blue Cohosh

Chandrasekhar, K and G. H. Sarma. 1974. "Observations on the Effect of Low and High Doses of *Caulophyllum* on the Ovaries and the Consequential Changes in the Uterus and Thyroid in Rats." *Journal of Reproduction and Fertility* 38(1):236–37.

Flom, M. S., R. W. Doskotch, and J. L. Beal. 1967. "Isolation and Characterization of Alkaloids from *Caulophyllum thalictroides.*" *J Pharm Sci.* 56(11):1515–17.

Olin, B. R. (Ed.). 1992. "Blue cohosh." *The Lawrence Review of Natural Products* October:1–2.

Woldemariam, T. Z., J. M. Betz, and P. J. Houghton. 1997. "Analysis of Aporphine and Quinolizidine Alkaloids from *Caulophyllum thalictroides* by Densitometry and HPLC." *J. Pharm. Biomed. Anal.* 15(6):839–43.

Boldo

Bastien, J. W. 1987. *Healers of the Andes— Kallaway Herbalists and Their Medicinal Plants.* Salt Lake City: University of Utah Press.

ESCOP. 1996. "*Boldo Folium.*" In *ESCOP Monographs on the Medicinal Use of Plant Drugs* (Vol. 1). Exeter, England: ESCOP Secretariat.

Gotteland, M., J. Espinoza, B. Cassels, and H. Speisky. 1995. "Effect of a Dry Boldo Extract on Oro-Cecal Intestinal Transit in Healthy Volunteers." *Rev. Med. Chil.* 123(8):955–960. (in Spanish).

Borage

Awang, D. V. C. 1990. "Borage." *Canadian Pharmaceutical Journal* 123:121–26.

Janick, J., J. E. Simon, J. Quinn and N. Beaubaire. 1989. "Borage: A Source of Gamma-Linolenic Acid." In L. E. Craker and J. E. Simon, (Eds.) *Herbs, Spices, and Medicinal Plants: Recent Advances in Botany, Horticulture, and Pharmacology* (Vol. 4). Binghamton, NY: Haworth Press.

Broom

Olin, B. R. (Ed.) 1989. "Broom." *The Lawrence Review of Natural Products* September:1–2.

Burdock

Bever, B. O., and G.R. Zahnd. 1979. "Plants with Oral Hypoglycemic Action." *Quarterly Journal of Crude Drug Research* 17:139–96.

Chandler, F. and F. Osborne. 1997. "Burdock." *Canadian Pharmaceutical Journal* 130(5):46–49.

Calendula

Della Loggia, R. et al. 1994. "The Role of Triterpenoids in the Topical Anti-Inflammatory Activity of *Calendula officinalis* Flowers." *Planta Medica* 60: 516–20.

ESCOP. 1996. "*Calendulae flos.*" In *ESCOP Monographs on the Medicinal Use of Plant Drugs* (Vol. 1). Exeter, England: ESCOP Secretariat.

Olin, B. R. (Ed.). 1995. "Calendula." *Lawrence Review of Natural Products. January.*

Patrick, K. F. M. et al. 1996. "Induction of Vascularization by an Aqueous Extract of the Flowers of *Calendula officinalis* L., the European Marigold." *Phytomedicine* 3(1):11–18.

Cascara Sagrada

Tyler, V. E., L. R. Brady, and J. E. Robbers. 1988. *Pharmacognosy* (9th ed.). Philadelphia: Lea & Febiger.

Cat's-Claw

Aquino, R. et al. 1991. "Plant Metabolites, New Compounds, and Anti-Inflammatory Activity of *Uncaria tomentosa.*" *Journal of Natural Products* 54(2):453–59.

Duke, J. 1994. "Una de gato." *The Business of Herbs. May/June.*

Jones, K. 1995. *Cat's-Claw—Healing Vine of Peru.* Seattle: Sylvan Press.

Rizzi, R. et al. 1993. "Mutagenic and Antimutagenic Activities of *Uncaria tomentosa* and Its Extracts." *Journal of Ethnopharmacology* 38:63–67.

Stuppner, H., et al. 1993. "A Differential Sensitivity of Oxindole Alkaloids to Normal and Leukemic Cell Lines." *Planta Medica* 59 (Supplement):583.

Wagner, H. et al. 1985. "Die Alkaloide von *Uncaria tomentosa* und ihre Phagozytosesteigernde Wirkung." *Planta Medica* 51: 419–23.

Cayenne

Palevitch, D. and L. Craker."Nutritional and Medical Importance of Red Pepper (*Capsicum* spp.)." *Journal of Herbs, Spices & Medicinal Plants* 3(2): 55–83.

Celery

Breiteneder, H. et al. 1995. "Molecular Characterization of Api g 1, the Major Allergen of Celery (*Apium graveolens*), and Its Immunological and Structural Relationships to a Group of 17-kDa Tree Pollen Allergens." *European Journal of Biochemistry* 233(2):484–89.

Duke, J. A. 1997. "An Herb a Day— Celery." *Business of Herbs* May/June:12–13.

Ljunggren, B. 1990. "Severe Phototoxic Burn Following Celery Ingestion." *Archives of Dermatology* 126(10):1334–36.

Chamomile

ESCOP. 1990. *Proposals for European Monographs* (Vol. 1). Bevrijdingslaan, Netherlands: European Scientific Cooperative for Phytotherapy.

Foster, S. 1996. "Chamomile (2nd ed.)." *Botanical Series* no. 307. Austin: American Botanical Council.

Salamon, L. 1992. "Chamomile in Slovakia." *The Herb, Spice and Medicinal Plant Digest* 10(1):1–4.

Chaparral

Katz, M. and F. Saibil. 1990. "Herbal Hepatitis: Subacute Hepatic Necrosis Secondary to Chaparral Leaf." *J. Clin. Gastroenterol.* 12(2):203–06.

Smart, C. R. et al. 1969. "An Interesting Observation on Nordihydroguaiaretic Acid (NSC 4291, NDGA) and a Patient with Malignant Melanoma—A Preliminary Report." *Cancer Chemotherapy Reports* (Part 1) 53:147.

Chickweed

Duke, J. A. 1992. *Handbook of Edible Weeds.* Boca Raton: CRC Press.

Rizk, A. M. 1986. *The Phytochemistry of the Flora of Qatar.* Doha, Qatar: The

Scientific and Applied Research Centre, University of Qatar.

Cranberry

Avorn, J. et al. 1994. "Reduction of Bacteriuria and Pyuria After Ingestion of Cranberry Juice." *Journal of the American Medical Association* 271(10): 751–54.

ESCOP. 1992. *Proposals for European Monographs* (Vol. 3). Bevrijdingslaan, Netherlands: European Scientific Cooperative for Phytotherapy.

Hobbs, C. 1989. "*Taraxacum Officinale*: A Monograph and Literature Review." In *Eclectic Dispensatory of Botanical Therapeutics* (Vol. 1). Portland: Eclectic Medical Publications.

Ofek, L., et al. 1991. "Anti-*Escherichia Coli* Adhesion Activity of Cranberry and Blueberry Juices." *New England Journal of Medicine* 324: 1599.

Zafari, D. et al. 1989. "Inhibitory Activity of Cranberry Juice on Adherence of Type 1 and Type P Fimbriated *Escherichia coli* to Eucaryotic Cells." *Antimicrobial Agents and Chemotherapy* 33:92–98.

Damiana

Elderidge, J. 1975. "Bush Medicines in the Exumas and Long Island Bahamas: A Field Study." *Economic Botany* 29(4):307–32.

Lloyd, J. U. 1904. "Damiana (The Mexican Tea). *Turnera aphrodisiaca.*" *The Pharmaceutical Review* 22:126–31.

Tyler, V. E. 1983. "History of an Herbal Hoax." *Pharmacy in History* 25(2):55.

Dandelion

ESCOP. 1996. "*Taraxaci folium* and *Taraxaci radix.*" In *ESCOP Monographs on the Medicinal Use of Plant Drugs* (Vol. 2). Exeter, England: ESCOP Secretariat.

Hobbs, C. 1989. "*Taraxacum officinale*: A Monograph and Literature Review." In *Eclectic Dispensatory of Botanical Therapeutics* (Vol. 1). Portland: Eclectic Medical Publications.

Neef, H. et al. 1996. "Platelet Anti-Aggregating Activity of *Taraxacum offici-*

nale Weber." *Phytotherapy Research* 10:S138–S140.

Devil's Claw

Chrubasik, S. et al. 1996. "Effectiveness of *Harpagophytum procumbens* in Treatment of Acute Low Back Pain." *Phytomedicine* 3(1):1–10.

Hebel, S. K. (Ed.). 1996. "Devil's Claw." *The Lawrence Review of Natural Products.* March:1–2.

Lanhers, M-C. et al. "Anti-Inflammatory and Analgesic Effects of an Aqueous Extract of *Harpagophytum procumbens.*" *Planta Medica* 58:117–23.

Watt, J. M. and M. G. Breyer-Brandwijk. 1962. *Medicinal and Poisonous Plants of Southern and Eastern Africa* (2nd ed.). Edinburgh: E. & S. Livingstone, Ltd.

Dong-quai

Belford-Cortney, R. 1993. "Comparison of Chinese and Western Uses of *Angelica sinensis.*" *Australian Journal of Medical Herbalism* 5(4):87–91.

Chang, H. M. and P. P. H. But (Eds.). 1986. *Pharmacology and Applications of Chinese Materia Medica* (Vol. 1). Singapore: World Scientific.

Li, L. et al. 1995. "A Study on Protein Metabolism in Nephrotic Patients Treated with Chinese Herbs." *Chung Hua Nei Ko Tsa Chih* 34(10):670–72.

Echinacea

Bauer R. and H. Wagner, 1991. "Echinacea Species as Potential Immunostimulatory Drugs." In *Economic and Medicinal Plant Research* (Vol. 5). Orlando: Academic Press.

Braunig, B. et al. 1992. "*Echinacea purpurea radix* for Strengthening the Immune Response in Flu-like Infections." *Zeitschrift fur Phytotherapie* 13:7–13.

Foster, S. 1991. *Echinacea: Nature's Immune Enhancer.* Rochester, VT: Healing Arts Press.

Melchart, D. et al. 1994. "Immunomodulation with Echinacea—

A Systematic Review of Controlled Clinical Studies." *Phytomedicine* 1: 245–54.

See, D. M. et al. 1997. "*In vitro* Effects of Echinacea and Ginseng on Natural Killer and Antibody-dependent Cell Cytotoxicity in Healthy Subjects and Chronic Fatigue Syndrome or Acquired Immunodeficiency Syndrome Patients." *Immunopharmacology* 35:229–35.

Elderberry

Elliman, W. 1994. "Elderberry, Flu Contrary." *Hadassah Magazine* December: 40–41.

Mumcuoglu, M. 1995. *Sambuco—Black Elderberry Extracts: A Breakthrough in the Treatment of Influenza.* Skokie: RSS Publishing, Inc.

Zakay-Rones, Z. et al. "Inhibition of Several Strains of Influenza Virus *in Vitro* and Reduction of Symptoms by an Elderberry Extract (*Sambucus nigra* L.) During an Outbreak of Influenza B Panama." *The Journal of Alternative and Complementary Medicine* 1(4):361–69.

Eleuthero

Farnsworth, N. R et al. 1985. "Siberian Ginseng (*Eleutherococcus senticosus*): Current Status as an Adaptogen." In *Economic and Medicinal Plant Research* (Vol. 1). Orlando: Academic Press.

Foster, S. 1996. "Siberian Ginseng, *Eleutherococcus senticosus.*" Botanical Series, no. 302. Austin: American Botanical Council.

Ephedra

Chen, K. K. 1974. "Half a Century of Ephedrine." *American Journal of Chinese Medicine* 2(4):359–65.

Dickinson, A. 1996. *FDA Food Advisory Committee Meeting on Ephedra-Containing Dietary Supplements—A Summary and Commentary.* Washington, DC: Council for Responsible Nutrition.

Kalix, P. 1991. "The Pharmacology of Psychoactive Alkaloids from Ephedra and Catha." *Journal of Ethnopharmacology* 32: 201–208.

Evening Primrose

Briggs, C. J. 1986. "Evening Primrose: *La Belle de Nuit,* The King's Cureall." *Canadian Pharmaceutical Journal* May: 249–54.

Horrobin, D. E. 1990 "Gamma Linolenic Acid." *Reviews in Contemporary Pharmacology* 1: 1–45.

Khoo, S. K. et al. 1990. "Evening Primrose Oil and Treatment of Premenstrual Syndrome." *Medical Journal of Australia* 153: 189–192.

Morse, P. F. et al. 1989. "A Meta-Analysis of Placebo-Controlled Studies of the Efficacy of Epogam in the Treatment of Atopic Eczema. Relationship Between Plasma Essential Fatty Acid Changes and Clinical Response." *British Journal of Pharmacology* 121:75–90.

Eyebright

Harkiss, K. J. and P. Timmins. 1973. "Studies in the Scrophulariaceae Part VIII. Phytochemical Investigation of *Euphrasia officinalis.*" *Planta Medica* 23:324–27.

Sticher, O., and O. Salama. 1981. "Iridoid Glucosides from *Euphrasia rostkoviana.*" *Planta Medica* 42:122–23.

Fennel

Abdul-Ghani A. and R. Amin. 1988. "The Vascular Action of Aqueous Extracts of *Foeniculum vulgare* leaves." *Journal of Ethnopharmacology* 24(2–3):213–18.

Albert-Puleo, M. 1980. "Fennel and Anise as Estrogenic Agents." *Journal of Ethnopharmacology* 2(4):334–44.

ESCOP. 1996. "*Foeniculi fructus.*" In *ESCOP Monographs on the Medicinal Use of Plant Drugs* (Vol. 1). Exeter, England: ESCOP Secretariat.

Fenugreek

Ajabnoor, M. A. and A. K. Tilmisany. 1988. "Effect of *Trigonella foenum-graecum* on Blood Glucose Levels in Normal and Alloxan-Diabetic Mice." *Journal of Ethnopharmacology* 22:45–49.

Raghuram, T. C. et al. 1994. "Effect of Fenugreek Seeds on Intravenous Glucose Disposition in Non-insulin Dependent Diabetic Patients." *Phytotherapy Research* 8:83–86.

Sharma, R. D. et al. 1966. "Hypolipidaemic Effect of Fenugreek Seeds: A Chronic Study in Non-insulin Dependent Diabetic Patients." *Phytotherapy Research* 10:332–34.

Feverfew

Awang, D. V. C. 1989. "Feverfew." *Canadian Pharmaceutical Journal* 122(5): 266–70.

Awang, D. V. C. et al. 1991. Parthenolide Content of Feverfew (*Tanacetum parthenium*) Assessed by HPLC and H-NMR Spectroscopy." *Journal of Natural Products* 54(6): 1516–21.

De Weerdt C. J., H. P. R. Bootsma, and H. Hendricks. 1996. "Herbal Medicines in Migraine Prevention: Randomized Double-Blind Placebo-Controlled Crossover Trial of a Feverfew Preparation." *Phytomedicine* 3(3):225–30.

Foster, S. 1996. "Feverfew—*Tanacetum parthenium.*" *Botanical Series,* no. 310. Austin: American Botanical Council.

Johnson, E. S. et al. 1985. "Efficacy of Feverfew as a Prophylactic Treatment of Migraine." *British Medical Journal* 291: 569–73.

Murch, S. J., C. B. Simmons, and P. K. Saxena. 1997. "Melatonin in Feverfew and other Medicinal Plants." *The Lancet* 350 November 29:1598–99.

Murphy, J. et al. 1988. "Randomized, Double-Blind, Placebo-Controlled Trial of Feverfew in Migraine Prevention." *The Lancet* July 23:189–92.

Palevitch, D., G. Earon, and R. Carasso. 1997. "Feverfew (*Tanacetum parthenium*) as a Prophylactic Treatment for Migraine: A Double-Blind Placebo-Controlled Study." *Phytotherapy Research* 11(7):506–511.

Fo-ti

Grech, J. N. et. al. 1994. "Novel CA2+-

AtPase Inhibitors from the Dried Root of *Polygonum multiflorum.*" *Journal of Natural Products* 57(12): 1682–87.

Hong, C. Y. et al. 1994. "*Astragalus membranaceus* and *Polygonum multiflorum* Protect Rat Heart Mitochondria Against Lipid Peroxidation." *American Journal of Chinese Medicine* 22(1): 63–70.

Horikawa, K. et al. 1994. "Moderate Inhibition of Mutagenicity and Carcinogenicity of Benzo[a]purene, 1,6-dinitropyrene, and 3,9-dinitroflouranthene by Chinese Medicinal Herbs." *Mutagenesis* 9(6):523–26.

Garcinia

Greenwood, M. R. C. et al. 1981. "Effect of (—)-Hydroxycitrate on Development of Obesity in the Zucker Obese Rat." *American Journal of Physiology* 240:E72–E78.

Majeed, M. et al. 1994. *Citrin: A Revolutionary, Herbal Approach to Weight Management.* Burlingame, CA: New Editions Publishing.

Rao, R. N., and K. K. Sakariah. 1988. "Lipid-Lowering and Antiobesity Effect of (—)Hydroxycitric Acid." *Nutrition Research* 8:209–212.

Sullivan, A. C. and R. K. Gruen. 1985. "Mechanisms of Appetite Modulation by Drugs." *Federation Proceedings* 44(1):139–44.

Garlic

Ali, M. and M. Thomson. 1995. "Consumption of a Garlic Clove a Day Could be Beneficial in Preventing Thrombosis." *Prostaglandins, Leukotrienes and Essential Fatty Acids* 53(5):211–12.

Foster, S. 1996. "Garlic—*Allium sativum.*" *Botanical Series* no. 311. Austin: American Botanical Council.

Koch, H. P and L. D. Lawson, (Eds.). 1995. *Garlic—The Science and Therapeutic Application of Allium sativum L. and Related Species* (2nd ed.). Baltimore: Williams & Wilkins.

Reuter, H. D. 1995. "*Allium sativum* and *Allium ursinum:* Part 2, Pharmacology and

Medicinal Application." *Phytomedicine* 2(1): 73–91.

Gentian

Hobbs, C. 1991. "Gentian—A Bitter Pill to Swallow." *Pharmacy in History* 33(3): 131–135.

Olin, B. R. (Ed.). 1993. "Gentian." *Lawrence Review of Natural Products* April:1–2.

Rosseti, V. 1984. "Composition of *Gentiana lutea* L. Dried Roots Harvested at Different Altitudes." *Plantes Mdicinales et Phytothrapie* 18(1):15–23.

Ginger

Awang, D. V. C. 1992. "Ginger." *Canadian Pharmaceutical Journal* July: 309–11.

Bone, M. E. et al. 1990. "Ginger Root—A New Antiemetic. The Effect of Ginger Root on Postoperative Nausea and Vomiting after Major Gynecological Surgery." *Anesthesia* 45(8):669.

Grontved, A. et al. 1988. "Ginger Root Against Seasickness." *Acta Otolaryngol (Stockh)* 105:45–49.

Mowrey, D. B. and D. E. Clayson. 1982. "Motion Sickness, Ginger and Pyschophysics." *The Lancet* 20:655–667.

Sharma, I. et al. 1996. "Hypolidiaemic and Antiatherosclerotic Effects of *Zingiber officinale* in Cholesterol Red Rabbits." *Phytotherapy Research* 10(6): 517–18.

Wood, C. D. et al. 1988. "Comparison of Efficacy of Ginger with Various Antimotion Sickness Drugs." *Clinical Research Practices and Drug Regulatory Affairs* 6(2):129–36.

Yamahara, et. al. 1990. "Gastrointestinal Motility-Enhancing Effect of Ginger and its Active Constituents." *Chemical and Pharmaceutical Bulletin* 38(2):430–31.

Ginkgo

DeFeudis, E. V. 1991. Ginkgo biloba *Extract (EGb 761): Pharmacological Activities and Clinical Applications.* Amsterdam: Elsevier.

Foster, S. 1996. "*Ginkgo biloba.*" *Botanical Series* no. 304. Austin: American Botanical Council.

Funfgeld, E. W. (Ed.). 1988. *Rokan* (Ginkgo biloba), *Recent Results in Pharmacology and Clinic.* Berlin: Springer-Verlag.

Kanowski, S. et al. 1996. "Proof of Efficacy of the *Ginkgo biloba* Special Extract EGb 761 in Outpatients Suffering from Mild to Moderate Primary Degenerative Dementia of the Alzheimer Type or Multi-Infarct Dementia." *Pharmacopsychiatry* 29:47–56.

Kleijnen, J. and P Knipschild. 1992. "*Ginkgo biloba* for Cerebral Insufficiency." *British Journal of Clinical Pharmacology* 34:352–58.

Le Bars, P. L. et al. 1997. "A Placebo-Controlled, Double-Blind, Randomized Trial of an Extract of *Ginkgo biloba* for Dementia." *Journal of the American Medical Association* 278:1327–32.

Sohn, M. and R. Sikora. 1991. "*Ginkgo biloba* Extract in the Therapy of Erectile Dysfunction." *Journal of Sex Education and Therapy* 17:53–61.

Ginseng

Foster, S. 1996. "Asian Ginseng, *Panax ginseng.*" *Botanical Series* no. 303. Austin: American Botanical Council.

_____. 1996. "American Ginseng, *Panax quinquefolius.*" *Botanical Series* no. 308. Austin: American Botanical Council.

Hu, S. Y. 1976. "The Genus *Panax* (Ginseng) in Chinese Medicine." *Economic Botany* 30:11–28.

_____. 1977. "A Contribution to Our Knowledge of Ginseng." *American Journal of Chinese Medicine* 5:1–23.

Le Gal, M., P. Cathebras and K. Strby. 1996. "Pharmaton Capsules in the Treatment of Functional Fatigue: A Double-Blind Study Versus Placebo Evaluated by a New Methodology." *Phytotherapy Research* 10(1):49–53.

Ng, T. B. and H. W. Yeung. 1986. "Scientific Basis of the Therapeutic Effects of Ginseng." In *Folk Medicine, The Art and the Science.* Washington, DC: American Chemical Society.

Shibata, S., O. Tanaka, J. Shoji, and H.

Saito. 1985. "Chemistry and Pharmacology of *Panax.*" In *Economic and Medicinal Plant Research* (Vol. 1). Orlando: Academic Press.

Goldenseal

Combie, J., T. E. Nugent, and T. Tobin. 1982. "Inability of Goldenseal to Interfere with the Detection of Morphine in Urine." *Equine Veterinary Science* January/February:16–21.

Foster, S. 1989. "Goldenseal—Masking of Drug Tests from Fiction to Fallacy: An Historical Anomaly." *HerbalGram* 21: 7, 35.

_____. 1996. "Goldenseal *Hydrastis canadensis.*" *Botanical Series* no. 309. Austin: American Botanical Council.

Genest, K., and D. W. Hughes. 1969. "Natural Products in Canadian Pharmaceuticals IV *Hydrastis Canadensis.*" *Canadian Journal of Pharmaceutical Science* 4:41–45.

Palmary, M., M. F. Cometa, and M. G. Leone. 1996. "Further Studies on the Adrenolytic Activity of the Major Alkaloids from *Hydrastis canadensis* L. on Isolated Rabbit Aorta." *Phytotherapy Research* 10:S47–S49.

Gotu Kola

Divan, P. V. et al. 1991. "Anti-Anxiety Profile of Manduk Parni (*Centella asiatica*) in Animals." *Fitoterapia* 62:3, 253–57.

Kartnig, T. 1988. "Clinical applications of *Centella asiatica* (L.) Urb." In *Herbs, Spices, and Medicinal Plants—Recent Advances in Botany, Horticulture and Pharmacology* (Vol. 3). Phoenix: Oryx Press.

Morisset, R. et al. 1987. "Evaluations of the Healing Activity of Hydrocotyle Tincture in the Treatment of Wounds." *Phytotherapy Research* 1(3):117–21.

Nalini, N. et al. 1992. "Effect of *Centella asiatica* Fresh Leaf Aqueous Extract on Learning and Memory and Biogenic Amine Turnover in Albino Rats." *Fitoterapia* 63(3):232–37.

Grapeseed

Bombardelli, E. and P. Morazzoni. 1995. "*Vitis vinifera.*" *Fitoterapia* 66(4):291–317.

Foster, S. 1997. "Grapeseed Extract." *Health Foods Business* April: 42–43.

Hawthorn

Hamon, N. W. 1988. "Herbal medicine: Hawthorns (Genus *Crataegus*)." *Canadian Pharmaceutical Journal* 121:708–09, 724.

Hobbs, C., and S. Foster. 1989. "Hawthorn: A Literature Review." *HerbalGram* 22:18–33.

Lloyd, J. U. 1921. "A Treatise on *Crataegus.*" *Drug Treatise No. 29.* Cincinnati: Lloyd Brothers Pharmacists.

Hops

ESCOP. 1996. "*Lupuli Flos.*" In *ESCOP Monographs on the Medicinal Use of Plant Drugs* (Vol. 4). Exeter, England: ESCOP Secretariat.

Horehound

Schlemper, V. et al. 1996. "Antispasmodic Effects of Hydroalcoholic Extract of *Marrubium vulgare* on Isolated Tissues." *Phytomedicine* 3(2):211–16.

Telek, E. et al. 1997. "Chemical tests with *Marrubium* species. Official data on *Marubii herba* in Pharmacopoeia Hungarica VII." *Acta Pharm. Hung.* 67(1):31–37. (In Hungarian).

Horse Chestnut

Bombardelli, E. and P. Morazzoni. 1996. "Aesculus hippocastanum." *Fitoterapia* 62(6):483–511.

Calabrese, C. and P. Preston. 1993. "Report of the Results of a Double-Blind, Randomized, Single-Dose Trial of a Topical 2% Escin Gel versus Placebo in the Acute Tratment of Experimentally-Induced Hematoma in Volunteers." *Planta Medica* 59:394–97.

Diehm, C. et al. 1996. Comparison of Leg Compression Stocking and Oral Horse Chestnut Seed Extract in Therapy in Patients with Chronic Venous Insufficiency." *The Lancet* 347:292–94.

Horsetail

Hamon, N. W. and D. V. C. Awang. "Horsetail." *Canadian Pharmaceutical Journal* September:399–401.

Henderson, J. A. et al. 1952. The Antithiamine Action of *Equisetum.*" *Journal of the American Veterinary Medicine Association* June:375–78.

Olin, B. R. (Ed.). 1991. "Horsetail." *Lawrence Review of Natural Products* October:1–2.

Hyssop

Gollapudie, S. et al. 1995. "Isolation of a Previously Unidentified Polysaccharide (MAR-10) from *Hyssop officinalis* that Exhibits Strong Activity Against Human Immunodeficiency Virus. *Biochemical and Biophysical Research Communications (1):145–51).*

Hagemann, R. C. et al. (Eds). 1996. "Hyssop." *The Lawrence Review of Natural Products* September:1–2.

Kreis, W. et al.1990. "Inhibition of HIV Replication by *Hyssopus officinalis* Extracts." *Antiviral Research* 14(6):323–37.

Juniper

ESCOP. 1997. "*Juniperi Fructus.*" In *ESCOP Monographs on the Medicinal Use of Plant Drugs (Vol. 3.* Exeter, England: ESCOP Secretariat.

Kava-kava

Lebot, V. et al. 1992. *Kava—The Pacific Drug.* New Haven, CT: Yale University Press.

Lehmann, E. et al. 1996. "Efficacy of a Special Kava Extract (*Piper methysticum)* in Patients with States of Anxiety, Tension, and Excitedness of Non-Mental Origin—A Double-Blind, Placebo-Controlled Study of Four Weeks Treatment." *Phytomedicine,* 3(2):113–19.

Kudzu

Foster, S. 1994. "Kudzu Monograph." *Quarterly Review of Natural Medicine* Winter:303–08.

Keung, W. M. and B. L. Vallee 1993. "Daidzin and Daidzein Suppress Free-choice Ethanol Intake by Syrian Golden Hamsters." *Proceedings of the National Academy of Sciences USA* 90:10008–12.

Shukla, S. et al. 1996. "Protective Action of Butanolic Extract of *Pueraria tuberosa* DC Against Carbon Tetrachloride-Induced Hepatotoxicity in Adult Rats." *Phytotherapy Research* 10(7):608–09.

Zhou, Y. P. 1984. "Recent Progress on the Pharmacological Research and Clinical Applications of *Pueraria* Roots." *Chinese J. Integr. Trad. Western Med.* 11:699–702.

Lemon Balm

Wobling, R. H. and K. Leonhardt. 1994. "Local therapy of *Herpes simplex* with dried extract from *Melissa officinalis.*" *Phytomedicine* 1(1): 25–31.

Lemon Grass

Carlini, E. A. et al. 1986. "Pharmacology of Lemongrass (*Cymbopogon citratus* Stapf). I. Effects of Teas Prepared from the Leaves on Laboratory Animals." *Journal of Ethnopharmacology* 17(1):37–64.

Leite, J. R. et al. 1986. "Pharmacology of Lemongrass (*Cymbopogon citratus* Stapf). III. Assessment of Eventual Toxic, Hypnotic and Anxiolytic Effects on Humans." *Journal of Ethnopharmacology* 17(1):75–83.

Weniger, B. and L. Robineau. 1988. *Elements for a Caribbean Pharmacopeia.* Havana: TRAMIL.

Licorice

Hayashi, H. et al. 1993. "Distribution Pattern of Saponins in Different Organs of *Glycrrhiza glabra.*" *Planta Medica* 59:351–53.

Kimura, Y. et al. 1993. "Effects of Flavonoids from Licorice Roots (*Glycrrhiza inflata* Bat.) on Arachidonic Acid Metabolism and Aggregation in Human Platelets." *Phytotherapy Research* 7:341–47.

Nielsen, L. and R. S. Pederson. 1984. "Life-Threatening Hypokalaemia Caused by Licorice Ingestion." *The Lancet* 2:1305.

Marshmallow

Ninov, S. et al. 1992. Constituents of *Althaea officinalis* var. 'Russalka' Roots." *Fitoterapia* 63:474.

Tomoda, M. et al. 1987. "Hypoglycemic Activity of Twenty Plant Mucilages and Three Modified Products." *Planta Medica* 53:8–12.

Milk Thistle

Foster, S. 1996. "Milk Thistle *Silybum marianum.*" *Botanical Series* no. 305. Austin: American Botanical Council.

Leng-Peschlow, E. and A. Strenge-Hesse. 1991. "The Milk Thistle (*Silybum marianum*) and Silymarin in Liver Therapy." *Phytotherapie* 12(5): 162–74.

Salmi, H. A. and S. Sarna. 1982. "Effect of Silymarin on Chemical, Functional, and Morphological Alterations of the Liver: A Double-Blind Controlled Study." *Scandanavian Journal of Gastroenterolology* 17:517–21.

Motherwort

Hu, S. Y. 1976. A Contribution to Our Knowledge of *Leonurus* L., *I-mu-ts'ao*, the Chinese Motherwort." *American Journal of Chinese Medicine* 4(3):219–37.

Kartig, T. et al. 1985. "Flavonoid-O-glycosides from the herb of *Leonurus cardiaca.*" *Journal of Natural Products* 48:494–507.

Kong, Y. C., et al. 1976. "Isolation of the Uterotonic Principle from *Leonurus artemisia*, the Chinese Motherwort. *American Journal of Chinese Medicine* 4(4):373–82.

Wang, Z. S. et al. 1988. The Therapeutic Effect of *Herba Leonuri* in the Treatment of Coronary Myocardial Ischemia. *Journal of Traditional Chinese Medicine* 8(2):103–06.

Mullein

McCutcheon, A. R. et al. 1995. "Antiviral Screening of British Columbian Medicinal Plants." *Journal of Ethnopharmacology* 49(2):101–10.

Mehrotra, R. et al. 1989. "Verbascoside: A New Luteolin Glycoside from *Verbascum thapsus. Journal of Natural Products* 52(3):640–43.

Olin, B. R. (Ed.). 1989. "Mullein." *The Lawrence Review of Natural Products* September:1.

Neem

National Academy of Sciences. 1992. *Neem: A Tree for Solving Global Problems.* Washington, DC: National Academy Press.

Tewari, D. N. 1992. *Monograph on Neem.* Derha Dun, India: R. O. Singh Gahlot.

Nopal

Munoz de Chavez, M. et al. 1995. "The Nopal: A Plant of Manifold Qualities." *World Review of Nutrition and Diet* 77:109–34.

Palevitch, D., G. Earon, and I. Levin. 1993. "Treatment of Benign Prostatic Hypertrophy with *Opuntia ficus-indica* (L.) Miller." *Journal of Herbs Spices and Medicinal Plants* 2(1):45–49.

Olive Leaf

Keville, K. 1997. "The Herb Report—Olive." *The American Herb Association Newsletter* 13(4):3–5.

Parsley

Simon, J. E. and J. Quinn. 1988. "Characterization of Essential Oil of Parsley." *Journal of Agricultural and Food Chemistry* 36:467–72.

Zhgen, G. et al. 1992. "Myrsiticin: A Potentent Cancer Chemopreventive Agent from Parsely Leaf Oil." *Journal of Agricultural and Food Chemistry* 40:107–110.

Passionflower

ESCOP. 1997. "*Passiflora herba.*" In *ESCOP Monographs on the Medicinal Use of Plant Drugs* (Vol. 4). Exeter, England: ESCOP Secretariat.

Foster, S. 1991. "The Passionflowers." *The Herb Companion* August/September: 18–23.

Olin, B. R. (Ed.). 1989. "Passion Flower." *The Lawrence Review of Natural Products* May:1–2.

Speroni, E. and A. Minghetti. 1988. "Neuropharmacological Activity of Extracts from *Passiflora incarnata.*" *Planta Medica* 54:488–91.

Pau d'arco

Awang, D. V. C. et al. 1994. "Naphthoquionone Constituents of Commercial Lapacho/Pau D'Arco/Taheebo Products." *Journal of Herbs, Spices, and Medicinal Plants* 2(4):27–43.

Block, J. B. et al. 1974. "Early Clinical Studies with Lapachol." *Cancer Chemotherapy Reports.* Part 2, 4(4):27–28.

Jones, K. 1995. *Pau d'Arco.* Rochester, VT: Healing Arts Press.

Oswald, E. H. 1993/94. "Lapacho." *British Journal of Phytotherapy* 3(3):112–17.

Peppermint

ESCOP. 1997. "*Menthae Piperitae Aetheroleum* and *Menthae Piperitae Folium.*" In *ESCOP Monographs on the Medicinal Use of Plant Drugs* (Vol. 3). Exeter, England: ESCOP Secretariat.

Foster, S. 1996. "Peppermint—*Mentha piperita.*" *Botanical Series* no. 306. Austin: American Botanical Council.

Rees, W. D. W., B. K. Evans, and J. Rhodes. 1979. "Treating Irritable Bowel Syndrome with Peppermint Oil." *British Medical Journal* October 6:835–36.

Somerville, K. W., C. R. Richmond, and G. D. Bell. 1984. "Delayed Release of Peppermint Oil Capsules (Colpermin) for the Spastic Colon Syndrome: A Pharmacokinetic Study." *British Journal of Clinical Pharmacology* 18: 638–40.

Steam, S. 1801. *The American Herbal.* Walpole, NH: Thomas and Thomas.

Plantain

Burnham, T. H. (Ed.). 1988. "Plantain." *The Lawrence Review of Natural Products* January:1–4.

Murai, M. et al. 1995. "Phenylethanoids in the Herbs of *Plantago lanceolata* and Inhibitory Effect of Arachidonic Acid-Induced Mouse Ear Edema." *Planta Medica* 61:479–80.

Samuelsen, A. B. et al. 1995. "Isolation and Partial Characterization of Biologically Active Polysaccharides from *Plantago major* L. *Phytotherapy Research* 9:211–18.

Prickly Ash

Bowen, J. M. et al. 1996. "Neuromuscular Effects of Toxins Isolated from Southern Prickly Ash (*Zanthoxylum clava-herculis*) bark." *American Journal of Veterinary Research* 57(8):1239–44.

Fish, F. et al. 1975. "Alkaloids and Coumarins from North American Zanthoxylum species." *Lloydia* 38(3):268–270.

Psyllium

ESCOP. 1996. *Plantaganis Ovatae Semen* and *Plantaganis Ovatae Testa.* In *ESCOP Monographs on the Medicinal Use of Plant Drugs* (Vol. 2). Exeter, England: ESCOP Secretariat.

Sprecher, D. L. et al. 1993. "Efficacy of psyllium in reducing serum cholesterol levels in hypercholesterolemic patients on high- or low-fat diets." *Annals of Internal Medicine* 119(7):545–54.

Pygeum

Cunningham, M., A. B. Cunningham, and U. Schippmann. 1997. *Trade in* Prunus africana *and the Implementation of CITES.* Munster: German Federal Agency for Nature Conservation.

Burnham, T. H. (Ed.). 1988. "Pygeum." *The Lawrence Review of Natural Products* January:1–2.

Raspberry Leaves

Bamford, D. S. et al. 1970. "Raspberry Leaf Tea: A New Aspect to an Old Problem." *British Journal of Pharmacology* 40:161–162P.

Briggs, C. J. and K. Briggs. 1997. "Raspberry." *Canadian Pharmaceutical Journal* April:41–43.

Red Clover

Aldercreutz, H. 1995. "Phytoestrogens: Epidemiology and a Possible Role in

Cancer Protection." *Environmental Health Perspectives* 103(7):103–12.

Aldercretz, H. and W. Mazur. 1997. "Phyto-oestrogens and Western Diseases." *Annals of Medicine* (2):95–120.

Cassady, J. M. et al. 1988. "Use of Mammalian Cell Culture Benzo(a)pyrene Metabolism Assay for the Detection of Potential Anticarcinogens from Natural Products: Inhibition of Metabolism by Biochanin A, an Isoflavone from *Trifolium pratense* L." *Cancer Research* 48: 6257–61.

Duke, J. A. 1990. "Red clover." *Business of Herbs* September/October:8–9.

Yanagihara, K. et al. 1993. "Antiproliferative effects of Isoflavones on Human Cell Cancer Lines Established from the Gastrointestinal Tract." *Cancer Research* 53: 5815–21.

Reishi

Hobbs, C. 1995. *Medicinal Mushrooms: An Exploration of Tradition, Healing and Culture.* Santa Cruz, CA: Botanica Press.

Rhubarb

Foust, C. M. 1992. *Rhubarb—The Wonderous Drug.* Princeton, NJ: Princeton University Press.

Hu, S. L. (Ed.). 1990. *Abstracts of the First International Symposium on Rhubarb.* Beijing: State Administration of Traditional Chinese Medicine.

Marshall, D. E. 1988. *A Bibliography of Rhubarb and Rheum Species.* USDA, NAL, ARS, Bibliographies and Literature of Agriculture. No. 62.

Rosemary

Haraguchi, H. et al. 1995. "Inhibition of lipid peroxidation and superoxide generation biditerpenoids from *Rosmarinus officinalis.*" *Planta Medica* 61(4):333–36.

Hjorther, A. B. et al. 1997. "Occupational Allergic Contact Dermatitis from Carnosol, a Naturally-Occurring Compound Present in Rosemary." *Contact Dermatitis* 37(3):99–100.

Huang, M.T. et al. 1994. "Inhibition of Skin Tumorigenesis by Rosemary and its Constituents Carnosol and Ursolic Acid." *Cancer Research* (3):701–O8

Offord, E.A. et al. 1995. "Rosemary Components Inhibit Benzo[a]pyrene-Induced Genotoxicity in Human Bronchial Cells." *Carcinogenesis* 16(9):2057–62.

Sage

ESCOP. 1996. "*Salvia folium.*" In *ESCOP Monographs on the Medicinal Use of Plant Drugs* (Vol. 2). Exeter, England: ESCOP Secretariat.

Sarsaparilla

Hobbs, C. 1988. "Sarsaparilla—A Literature Review." *HerbalGram* 17:1, 10–15.

Suh, H. W. et al. 1996. "Antinociceptive Effects of Smilaxin B Administered Intracerebroventricularly in the Mouse." *Planta Medica* 62:141–45.

Saw Palmetto

Braeckman, J., J. Bruhwyler, K. Vandekerckhove, and J. Gczy. 1997. "Efficacy and Safety of the Extract of *Serenoa repens* in the Treatment of Benign Prostatic Hyperplasia: The Therapeutic Equivalence Between Twice and Once Daily Dosage Forms." *Phytotherapy Research* 11(8):558–563.

Carraro, J-C. et al. 1996. "Comparison of Phytotherapy (Permixon) With Finasteride in the Treatment of Benign Prostate Hyperplasia: A Randomized International Study of 1,098 Patients." *The Prostate* 29:213–40.

Champault, G. et al. 1984. "The Medical Treatment of Prostatic Adenoma—A Controlled Study: PA-109 versus Placebo in 110 Patients." *Annals of Urology* 6: 407–10.

Hale, E. M. 1898. *Saw Palmetto.* Philadelphia: Boericke & Tafel.

Schisandra

Ip, S. P. et al. 1996. "Effect of a lignan-enriched extract of *Schisandra chinensis* on aflatoxin B1 and cadmium chloride-induced hepatotoxicity in rats." *Pharmacology and Toxicology* 78(6):413–16.

Ko, K. M., et al. 1995. "Effect of a Lignan-Enriched *Fructus Schisandrae* Extract on Hepatic Glutathione Status in Rats: Protection Against Carbon Tetrachloride Toxicity. *Planta Medica* 61(2):134–37.

Lu, H., and G. T. Liu. 1992. "Anti-oxidant activity of dibenzocyclooctene lignans isolated from Schisandraceae." *Planta Medica* 53(4):311–13.

Nishiyama, N., Y. L. Wang, and H. Saito. 1995. "Beneficial effects of S-113m, a novel herbal prescription, on learning impairment model in mice." *Biol. Pharm. Bull.* 11:1498–503.

Senna

ESCOP. 1997. "*Sennae folium.*" In *ESCOP Monographs on the Medicinal Use of Plant Drugs* (Vol. 5). Exeter, England: ESCOP Secretariat.

ESCOP. 1997. "*Sennae fructus acutifoliae.*" In *ESCOP Monographs on the Medicinal Use of Plant Drugs* (Vol. 5). Exeter, England: ESCOP Secretariat.

Leng-Preschlow, E. (Ed.). 1992. "Senna and Its Rational Use." *Pharmacology* 44(S1): 1–52.

Shepherd's Purse

Kuroda, K. and T. Kaku. 1969. "Pharmacological and Chemical Studies on the Alcohol Extract of *Capsella bursa-pastoris.*" *Life Sciences* 8:151–55.

Vermathen, M. and H. Glasl. 1993. "Effect of the Herb Extract of *Capsella bursa-pastoris* on Blood Coagulation." *Planta Medica* 59S:A670.

Skullcap

Anon. 1985. "Scullcap Substitution." *HerbalGram* Fall:3.

Huxtable, R. J. 1992. 1992. "The Myth of Beneficent Nature: The Risks of Herbal Preparations." *Annals of Internal Medicine* 117(2):165–66.

Leander, S. and L. Skogstrom. 1991. "Natural Medicine Can Cause Liver Damage." *Aftenposten,* November 6.

Slippery Elm

Foster, S. 1991. "Slippery Elm." *Business of Herbs* March/April.

Tyler, V. and S. Foster. 1996. "Herbs and Phytomedicinal Products." In *Handbook of Nonprescription Drugs* (11th ed.). Washington, DC: American Pharmaceutical Association.

St.-John's-Wort

Awang, D. V. C. 1991. "St. John's Wort." *Canadian Pharmaceutical Journal* 124:33–35.

Harrer, G. and H. Sommer. 1994. "Treatment of Mild/Moderate Depressions with *Hypericum.*" *Phytomedicine* 1(1):3–8.

Linde, K. et al. 1996. "St. John's Wort for Depression–An Overview and Meta-Analysis of Randomized Clinical Trials." *British Medical Journal* 313:253–58.

Suzuki, O. et al. 1984. "Inhibition of Monoamine Oxidase by Hypericin." *Planta Medica* 50:272–74.

Stinging Nettle

Belaiche, P. and O. Lievoux. "Clinical Studies on the Palliative Treatment of Prostatic Adenoma with Extract of *Urtica* Root." *Phytotherapy Research* 5: 267–69.

Gansser, D. and G. Spiteller. 1995. "Aromatase inhibitors form *Urtica dioica* Roots." *Planta Medica* 61:138–40.

Hirano, T. et al. 1994. "Effects of Stinging Nettle Root Extracts and Their Steroidal Components on the Na+, K+-ATPase of the Benign Prostatic Hyperplasia." *Planta Medica* 60:30–33.

Hyrb, D. J. et al. 1995. "The Effects of Extracts of the Roots of the Stinging Nettle (*Urtica dioica*) on the Interaction of SHBG with its Receptor on Human Prostatic Membranes." *Planta Medica* 61:31–32.

Patten, G. 1993. "*Urtica.*" *Australian Journal of Medical Herbalism* 5(1):5–13.

Tea Tree

Bassett, I. B. et al. 1990. "A Comparative Study of Tea Tree Oil Versus

Benzoylperoxide in the Treatment of Acne." *Medical Journal of Australia* 153(8): 455–58.

Buck, D. S. et al. 1994. "Comparison of Two Topical Preparations for the Treatment of Onychomycosis: *Melaleuca alternifolia* (Tea Tree) Oil and Clotrimazole." *The Journal of Family Practice* 38(6):601–05.

Carson, C. E. et al. 1995. "Susceptibility of Methicillin-Resistant *Staphylococcus aureus* to the Essential Oil of *Melaleuca alternifolia*." Journal of Antimicrobial Chemotherapy 38(6):421–24.

Foster, S. 1994. "Tea Tree and Its Relatives." *The Herb Companion* February/March:48–52.

Thyme

Ernst, E., R. März, and C. Sieder. 1997. "A Controlled Multi-Centre Study of Herbal Versus Synthetic Secretolytic Drugs for Acute Bronchitis." *Phytomedicine* 4(4):287–93.

Haraguchi, H. et al. 1996. "Antiperoxidative Components in *Thymus vulgaris*." *Planta Medica* 62(3): 217–21.

Turmeric

Ammon, H. P. T. and M. A. Wahl. 1991. "Pharmacology of *Curcuma longa*." *Planta Medica* 57:1–7.

Blumenthal, B. 1996. "From Curry to the Curious Curcuminoids." *Whole Foods* July:78–82.

McClatchey, W. 1993. "Traditional Uses of *Curcuma longa* (Zingiberaceae) in Rotuma." *Economica Botany* 47(3):291–96.

Rajakrishman, V., V. P. Menon, and K. N. Rajashekaran. 1998. "Protective Role of Curcumin in Ethanol Toxicity." *Phytotherapy Research* 12:55–56.

Selvam, R. et al. 1995. "The Antioxidant Activity of Turmeric (*Curcuma longa*). *Journal of Ethnopharmacology* 47:59–67.

Valerian

Chauffard, F. et al. 1982. "Detection of Mild Sedative Effects: Valerian and Sleep

in Man." *Experimentia* 37:622.

ESCOP. 1997. "Valerianae Radix." In *ESCOP Monographs on the Medicinal Use of Plant Drugs* (Vol. 4). Exeter, England: ESCOP Secretariat.

Foster, S. 1996. "Valerian—*Valeriana officinalis*." *Botanical Series,* no. 312. Austin: American Botanical Council.

Hobbs, C. 1989. "Valerian (*Valeriana officinalis*): A Literature Review." *HerbalGram* 21:19–34.

Houghton, R. J. 1988. "The Biological Activity of Valerian and Related Plants." *Journal of Ethnopharmacology* 22:121–42.

Leathwood, P. D., E Chauffard, E. Heck, and R Munoz-Box. 1982. "Aqueous Extract of Valerian Root (*Valeriana officinalis*) Improves Sleep Quality in Man, Reduces Sleep Latency to Fall Asleep in Man." *Pharmacology Biochemistry & Behavior* 17:65–71.

Schulz, V., R. Hänsel, and V. E. Tyler. 1998. "Valerian." In *Rational Phytotherapy: A Physician's Guide to Herbal Medicine.* Berlin: Springer.

Vitex

Bohnert, K.-J. and G. Hahn. 1990. "Phytotherapy in Gynecology and Obstetrics—*Vitex agnus-castus* (Chaste Tree)." *Acta Medica Emperica* 9: 494–502.

Brown, D. 1994. *Vitex agnus-castus* Clinical Monograph." *Quarterly Review of Natural Medicine* Summer:111–21.

Coeugniet, E., E. Elek, and R. Kuhnast. 1986. "Premenstrual Syndrome (PMS) and its Treatment." *Arztezeitschrift fur Naturheilverf* 27(9):619–22.

Dittmar, F. W. et al. 1992. "Premenstrual Syndrome (PMS): Treatment with a Phytopharmaceutical." *TIIY Gynakol* 5(1):60–68.

Feldmann, H. U., M. Albrecht, M. Lamertz, and K.-J. Bohnert. 1990. "The Treatment of Corpus Luteum Insufficiency and Premenstrual Syndrome: Experience in a Multicentre Study under Practice Conditions." *Hygne* 11(12):421.

Lauritzen, C. H. et al. 1997. "Treatment of Premenstrual Tension Syndrome with *Vitex agnus-castus*–Controlled, Double-blind Study Versus Pyridoxine." *Phytomedicine* 4(3):183–89.

White Oak

Foster, S. "White Oak." In *Benevolent Trees–A Woody Plants Herbal.* Unpublished manuscript.

Wild Yam

Araghiniknam, M. et al. 1996. "Antioxidant Activity of *Dioscorea* and dehydroepiandrosterone (DHEA) in Older Humans. *Life Sciences* 59:147–57.

Dentali, S. 1996. "More Yam To Chew On." *The American Herb Association Newsletter* 12:7.

Gaby, A. R. 1996. "Multi-level Yam Scam." *The American Herb Association Newsletter* 12:7.

Lloyd Brothers, Pharmacists, Inc. N.D. "A Treatise on *Dioscorea* and Sulphurous Acid. *Drug Treatise XIV*:1–9.

Smith, D. E. 1870. "*Dioscorea villosa.*" *Transactions of the Eclectic Medical Society of New York State* pp. 623–28.

Willow

Julkunen-Tiitto, R. and B. Meier. 1992. "The Enzymatic Decomposition of Salicin and Its Derivatives Obtained from Salicaceae Species." *Journal of Natural Products* 55(9):1204–12.

Tyler, V. and S. Foster. 1996. "Herbs and Phytomedicines." In *Handbook of Nonprescription Drugs* (11th ed.). Washington, DC: The American Pharmaceutical Association.

Witch Hazel

Korting, H. C. et al. 1995. "Comparative Efficacy of *Hamamelis* Distillate and Hydrocortisone." *European Journal of Clinical Pharmacology* 48(6):461–65.

Masaki, H., T. Atsumi, and H. Sakurai. 1995. "Protective Activity of Hamamelitannin on Cell Damage of Murine Skin Fibroblasts Induced by UVB Radiation." *Journal of Dermatological Science* 10(1):25–34.

Vennat, B. et al. 1988. "Tannins from *Hamamelis virginiana:* Identification of Proanthocyanidins and Hamamelitannin Quantification in Leaf, Bark, and Stem Extracts." *Planta Medica* 54:454–57.

Yellow Dock

Olin, B. R. 1992. "Yellow Dock." *The Lawrence Review of Natural Products* September:1.

Yucca

Bingham, R. et al. 1975. "Yucca Plant Saponin in the Management of Arthritis." *Journal of Applied Nutrition* 27:45–51.

Bingham, R. et al. 1978. "Yucca Plant Saponin in the Treatment of Hypertension and Hypercholesterolemia." *Journal of Applied Nutrition* 30:127–36.

Hayashi, K. et al. 1992. "Yucca Leaf Protein (YLP) Stops the Protein Synthesis in HSV-Infected Cells and Inhibits Virus Replication." *Antiviral Research* 17(4):323–33.

Lowe, J. A. and S. J. Kershaw. 1997. "The Ameliorating Effect of *Yucca schidigera* Extract on Canine and Feline Faecal Aroma." *Research in Veterinary Science* 63(1):61–66.

Uenobe, F., S. Nakamura, and M. Miyazawa. 1997. "Antimutagenic Effect of Resveratrol Against Trp-P-1." *Mutation Research* 373(2):197–200.

General References

Blumenthal, M. et al. (Eds.). 1998. S. Klein (Tr.). *German Commission E Therapeutic Monographs on Medicinals Herbs for Human Use.* Austin: American Botanical Council.

Bradly, P. R. (Ed.). 1992. *British Herbal*

Compendium (Vol. 1). Dorset, England: British Herbal Medicine Association.

Brown, D. 1996. *Herbal Prescriptions for Better Health*. Rocklin, CA: Prima.

Christopher, J. 1996. *School of Natural Healing*. Springville, UT: Christopher Publications.

Duke, James A. 1986. *Handbook of Medicinal Herbs*. Boca Raton: CRC Press.

Felter, H. W. and J. U. Lloyd. 1983. *King's American Dispensatory* (2 vols.). Portland: Eclectic Medical Publications.

Foster, S. 1993. *Herbal Renaissance*. Layton, UT: Gibbs Smith Publisher.

Foster, S. and J. A. Duke. 1990. *A Field Guide To Medicinal Plants: Eastern and Central North America*. Boston: Houghton Mifflin Co.

Foster, S. and C. X. Yue. 1992. *Herbal Emissaries: Bringing Chinese Herbs to the West*. Rochester, VT: Healing Arts Press.

Grieve, M. 1967.(1931). *A Modern Herbal* (2 vols.). New York: Hafner.

Kloss, J. 1939. *Back to Eden*. Coalmont, TN: Longview Publishing.

Lawson, L. D. and R. Bauer (Eds.). 1998. *Phytomedicine of Europe: Chemistry and Biological Activity*. ACS Symposium Series 691. Washington, DC: The American Chemical Society.

Leung, A. Y. and S. Foster. 1996. *Encyclopedia of Common Natural Ingredients Used in Food, Drugs, and Cosmetics* (2nd. ed.). New York: John Wiley & Sons.

Mabberly, D. J. 1997. *The Plant-Book* (2nd ed.). New York: Cambridge University Press.

McGuffin, M. et al. (Eds.). 1997. *American Herbal Product Association's Botanical Safety Handbook*. Boca Raton: CRC Press.

Newall, C. A., L. A. Anderson, and J. D. Phillipson. 1996. *Herbal Medicines: A Guide for Health-Care Professionals*. London: The Pharmaceutical Press.

Schulz, V., R. Hänsel, and V. E. Tyler. 1998. *Rational Phytotherapy: A Physician's Guide to Herbal Medicine*. Berlin: Springer.

Schilcher, H. 1997. *Phytotherapy in Paediatrics: Handbook for Physicians and Pharmacists*. Stuttgart: Medpharm Scientific Publishers.

Thompson, S. 1835. *New Guide to Health of Botanic Family Physician*. Boston: J. Q. Adams.

Tyler, V. E. 1993. *The Honest Herbal* (3rd ed.). Binghamtom, NY: Pharmaceutical Products Press.

_____. *Herbs of Choice–The Therapeutic Use of Phytomedicinals*. 1994. Binghamtom, NY: Pharmaceutical Products Press, 1994.

Tyler, V. and S. Foster. 1996. "Herbs and Phytomedicinal Products." In *Handbook of Nonprescription Drugs* (11th ed.). Washington, DC: American Pharmaceutical Association.

Weiss, R. F. 1988. *Herbal Medicine*. (Tr. A.R Meuss). Beaconsfield, England: Beaconsfield Publishers Ltd.

Witchl, M. 1994. *Herbal Drugs and Phytopharmaceuticals. (Tr. N. G. Bissett.)* Boca Raton: CRC Press.

Wren, R. C., revised by E. M. Williamson and E. J. Evans. 1988. *Potters New Cyclopedia of Botanical Drugs and Preparations (8th ed.)*. Essex: C. W. Daniel Co.

Glossary

anabolic activity: Metabolic action that converts simple substances into more complex compounds

antimutagen: Any substance that reduces, reverses, or counteracts the rate of spontaneous cell mutation or the action of a mutagen

antiphlogistic: Anti-inflammatory

aphrodisiac: Any substance that brings on sexual arousal

arthralgia: Joint pain

astringent: Any substance that causes tissues to contract when applied

autoimmune disease: Any disease arising from interference with or changes in the immune system's function; precise origin unknown

Ayurveda: India's ancient traditional system of medicine that uses hundreds of herbs for healing

bitters: bitter-tasting liquid mix of plant products; usually taken before meals to stimulate appetite and digestive juices

carbuncle: A large, staphlococcal, pus-filled skin infection with deep interconnecting pockets

carcinogenic: Able to start the development of cancer

cardiotonic: Of or pertaining to a substance that tends to increase the efficiency of the heart's contractions

carminative: A substance that relieves digestive gas and bloating

catarrh: Mucous membrane inflammation with discharge, especially involving air passages of the nose and trachea

chemopreventive: Substance that prevents cancer

contraindication: Something, such as a symptom or condition, that makes a treatment inadvisable

convalescence: A period of gradual recovery of strength and health after illness or weakness

decoction: Strong tea, usually made of woody or tough plant parts

dementia: A condition of deteriorated mentality, often with emotional apathy

detoxificiation: The process of removing a toxin or poison from the body

diaphoretic: Substance that increases sweating

diuresis: Increased urination

diuretic: Substance that increases urination

duodenal ulcer: A craterlike sore located where the stomach meets the small intestine

eczema: A superficial skin irritation of unknown cause; not a disease

edema: Swelling resulting from an abnormal accumulation of fluid in the spaces between the cells

elixir: A clear liquid containing alcohol, water, sweetener, and/or flavor used to deliver a medication

essential fatty acid: A polyunsaturated acid essential for the proper growth, maintenance, and functioning of the reproductive, glandular, and metabolic systems

essential oil: A concentrated, often aromatic oil distilled from plant material

expectorant: Substance that promotes expulsion of mucus from the respiratory tract

extract: Essential components drawn from a complex substance into a solution of alcohol, water, or other liquid

flatulence: Excessive digestive gas, and the expulsion of it

gastroenteritis: Inflammation of the stomach and intestine

gingivitis: Inflammation or disease of the gums

granulation: Soft fleshy projections that form during the healing process in a wound that does not heal normally

hypertension: High blood pressure

immunostimulant: Agent that stimulates the immune system

inflammation: The body's protective response to irritation or injury; includes redness, heat, pain, and swelling

laxative: A substance that gently stimulates the bowel to empty

lesion: A visible abnormality of the skin, such as a wound, boil, rash, or sore

libido: The internal drive for sex or pleasure

microcirculation: The flow of blood through the body's smaller vessels, especially capillaries

mucilage: A slick, slimy substance of various plants

permeable: Having pores or openings that allow substances to pass through

pharmacology: The study of the preparations, uses, and actions of drugs

photodermatitis: Increased skin sensitivity to light resulting in rapid sunburn, rash, or other symptoms

phytomedicine: Plant medicine

platelets: The smallest blood cells, primarily responsible for coagulation

poultice: Soft, moist plant pulp encased in cloth and applied to wound or irritation

respiration: Breathing

sedative: Calming agent

shingles: Painful, acute infection caused by reactivated chickenpox virus; afflicts mainly adults

stomatitis: Mouth inflammation caused by infection, chemicals, drugs, vitamin deficiency, or other conditions

styptic: Substance used to control bleeding

synergy: The process of two elements that work simultaneously to enhance each other

tannin: Acidic substance from bark and fruit of various plants used as an astringent

tincture: An extract of plant material in an alcohol-based solution

tonic: Substance that invigorates or restores

tuber: A fleshy underground plant stem

ulcer: A craterlike sore of the skin or mucous membrane

venous insufficiency: Decreased return of blood from the legs to the trunk of the body

vertigo: Dizziness

volatile oil: An oil that evaporates easily

Index